Weird Shit!

Sometimes in order to solve life's greatest existential conundrums one might need to engage in some really...

Weird Shit!

Janice Melmed

Published by
Kima Global Publishers
50 Clovelly Road,
Clovelly
7975
South Africa

ISBN 978-1-928513-12-4
eISBN 978-1-928513-13-1

Publisher's web site: www.kimabooks.com
Author's web site: www.janicemelmed.com

Table of Contents

Foreword

When Janice asked me to write the Foreword for Weird Shit!, I was both thrilled and humbled to do so. I first met Janice in 2003 and I watched the process slowly unfold as she struggled, against incredible odds, to find her way home. I am thrilled because this book is finally to be shared with you, the reader; I'm humbled because this is a book that will change lives of that I have no doubt.

As the founder of Inner Tuition SA, my journey of creating the courses started in 1997, slowly putting ideas on paper, and then struggling to share them with others in a way that made sense. I launched the same year under the name Wholism Healing which made very little sense, so in 2010 we renamed and relaunched as Inner Tuition. That is exactly what this journey is about – finding your own Inner Teacher. How does it work? I don't know, it simply does. Mainly because it is a perspective that is so simple, direct, and non-prescriptive, that it can be used by anyone, anywhere and in any situation. That's why we privately called it "the weird shit".

This book will change lives, of that I am sure. Many of the self-help books currently available ask, and assume, that the reader has a strong belief upon which they can build. Many people don't, or if they do, that belief is based on a wobbly foundation that cannot last the journey required. Janice has written a book which explains her faltering and floundering in an attempt to find that elusive light at the end of an endless, dark tunnel. Many promises were made by many people in different branches of medicine, therapists in many different modalities, many different suggestions, advice and instruction, many different philosophies, diets, exercises, treatments, rituals, and other more esoteric practices. She faithfully followed them all, giving each one her absolute trust. Very few helped.

Many others follow this same path and they get lost and increasingly confused and hopeless - and cynical. In this case however, this brave and insightful woman found her own way. With the help of Inner Tuition training courses, endless hours of discussion (when they were supposed to be listening to the trainer!), she put together all the knowledge she had gained from everyone, selected her own chosen nuggets of information, and she found her way. She looked inside herself and that was where the end of the tunnel was found – shining brightly.

Weird Shit!

I am writing this foreword dear reader, to encourage you to follow her story instead of her steps. Use her insights, or not, but they will help you to find your own way to your own answers. It gives me immense pleasure and pride to consider Janice a friend. I read this book in one sitting, one cold night in the middle of winter... I finished it at 3am. I was frozen stiff, but inside – I was glowing. This is the book I wanted to read, and I have wanted to encourage others to read. This book will be my Christmas gift, birthday gift and general just because gift for the next however long I have left. Enjoy finding out about Inner Tuition, and all the other byways that are covered in this story. Weird shit, indeed!

Margaret Holton, Founder of InnerTuition SA

Preface

Everyone has a story. Some stories are gloriously rich and full, tinged with excitement and adventure. Some are deep and meaningful, massively underscored by valour and maybe even heroics. Others are too terrible to countenance, and I can't even begin to go into this category because this is where everything that is wrong with our world resides. For the rest of us, our stories are shades of ordinary.

Please know that I mean no disrespect by saying you have an ordinary life. My personal goal for a major part of my life was to be ordinary. There is an enormous amount of comfort to be found in the ordinary day to day machinations of ordinary people. They live their lives according to the dictates of their specific group, class, race or community. Their behaviour is governed by the rules and rituals clearly established by the governing organisations of each particular group. They are watched over by either a beneficent, or a punitive spiritual order designed to inspire them to ordinariness and to keep them just fearful enough that they don't ever desire to be anything other than ordinary. Ah, the extraordinary ordinary masses!

For the most part, these ordinary people go about their business unperturbed by anything outside of their immediate needs' radius. They exist in total duality. Things are either black or white, good or bad, right or wrong, known or unknown, in or out. They are aware that there are shades of grey in the world and variations outside of their exacting beliefs and parameters, but the optimal word here is, outside. That which is not in, must be kept firmly and devoutly out.

They are born to loving families who instil in them the moral fibre and structure required to keep them on the straight and narrow. This is the path they are taught they need to follow in order to be rewarded, at the end of their lives, by whoever they believe the big guy in the sky is. This is the ultimate reward for a life well lived. They eat healthy, nutritionally balanced meals with just enough bad foods sprinkled in (often given, rather ironically, as a type of reward structure), to keep them strong, healthy and growing optimally; whilst allowing them a small titillation of their bad sides to keep life interesting. More importantly this feeds the fear that they could potentially turn bad one day so, in fact, this acts as an incentive to them to try harder to be good. If that sounds odd, then here's a simple example to illustrate.

- Set the goal – do well at school. The children have passed their exams.
- Reward good behaviour – they are treated to a bad food fest complete with bright blue milkshakes and deep-fried foods. This is so far outside of their meat and three veg staple that they feel amply recognised and rewarded and they feel proud of themselves.
- Instil fear and invoke guilt – remind them that this was an exception. A return to rules is immediately required to make sure that their bad side doesn't get out of control. That could lead to a collapse of all that they know to be true. They could end up feeling lethargic and get lazy about exercise. That in turn might make them feel sluggish leading to too much lying on the couch in front of the tv. That would lead to a decrease in brain power and the ultimate demise of their academic potential. They can no longer expect to get into good schools and become the exemplary citizens they were born to be. They could end up becoming drug dealers and living on park benches; all because of a burger, fries and blue milkshake.
- Assist in a return to order – get everyone up early the next morning for a group walk in the forest. If it was a particularly bad meal perhaps take along recyclable black bags to pick up trash at the same time. Encourage the children to run and skip and play in the sun and provide fresh wholesome snacks of fruit and nuts with low GI brown bread sandwiches and plentiful fresh, filtered water. These activities will restore them to goodness and they will have successfully neutralised the dangers inherent in the bad treat.
- Hold yourself up as an example to your people – tell your friends that your children achieved excellent results (good), that you rewarded them with a treat (bad), you neutralised the threat by rapid application of corrective measures (good). Since good won the day on the balanced scorecard of judgement, the world keeps turning, unblemished by your actions. You become someone to be admired, emulated even, and the ordinary people gain more power through this simple emulation. Extraordinary!!

You might see why I wanted to be ordinary. It paints a most wonderful picture of suburban bliss. Everyone knows what's expected of them, they are encouraged to meet expectations, and are rewarded accordingly. They are protected from themselves by rules and structures, and if that doesn't work, then they have a guy in the sky who can help them gain absolution and set them back on the right path.

Preface

No doubt, no fear, no confusion and everyone is happy. That, however, was not quite how my lot in life played out. I have spent decades trying to work out where I fit in, what I should be doing and the biggest question of all, "Who am I?" There's only one thing I know for certain … I didn't have a friggin'clue.

Part 1

Setting the scene

Chapter 1

The birthing conundrum

Have you ever thought, "Who am I?"or "Why am I here?" Well, those little nuggets have been in the background of my mind my entire life. One day I had a weird experience that left me completely stunned and started me on a journey of discovery that lasted almost twenty-five years. So, who am I? Let's find out!

I have things to share with you that I think you need to know. Important things, things that could change your life for the better. I learned this all the hard way, over so many years. I dragged it out, chewed it over and took my sweet-ass time to understand it. To try and save some dignity from my lengthy struggle, I've decided to share my story. If sharing my story helps even one person to find their truth in under twenty-five years, then maybe, just maybe, that struggle had a purpose. The alternative is that I'm just bloody slow on the uptake, not the sharpest tool in the shed if you know what I mean. So, stick with me please for the sake of my dignity. You don't have to believe a word I tell you. You can read all of this and write me off as a complete nutter. However, there is a very real possibility that I'm about to share with you the greatest truth you'll ever know, but you'll need to read on and decide for yourself... or not, you have the choice.

My earliest memory I uncovered during a session of hypnosis. I'd gone to a therapist to find out if I could find an underlying issue that was contributing to my weight problem. I was in my thirties, divorced with two children, gainfully employed and wondering what the fuck life was all about. It seemed to me that if I was ever going to find the man of my dreams (how can that be the highest goal, smacks hand to forehead), I would have to shape up a bit; but my body resisted all attempts to slim down. I'd read enough to know that therapy could be a useful tool so I set myself an agenda and signed up for three sessions with a hypnotherapist. I believed this to be the most time efficient manner to get to the bottom of the issue. I figured, one session to identify the root cause of the problem; a second one to formulate a strategy for correction/adjustments; and finally, a third to check in and see if anything further was needed and to wrap up with, hopefully, positive feedback from both sides. Anyone else spot the control issues?

Weird Shit!

Well you know what they say about the best laid plans of mice and men? Mother had always told me never to trust a man with a beard. My therapist, when he opened the door, was astonishingly hirsute, I'm talking Silverbacks in the mist on the mountains of Rwanda. I was so startled by the levels of his hairiness, that I blurted out this Mother-gem. He chuckled, seemed to find it amusing and ushered me inside, although he was probably thinking what an incredibly rude woman. My internal dialogue went as follows, "This is a dangerous situation. Really? What the heck, it's only hair. Let's give this go since I'm already here." Also, if the truth be told, I never really put that much stock in Mother's opinions anyway because she was… well she was… shall we say, a bit on the odd side. A lot of what she did and said was governed by what *they* were saying about her. She formed some very odd mannerisms to avoid *them* and *their* inevitable condemnation of her, and by extension of course, me. My childhood had been a delicate balancing act of trying to get by without rocking the boat, or poking the bear, or gaining the disapproving attentions of *them*. Once *they* were aroused, she tended to lash out and was hard to placate. She also had a memory like an elephant and never, ever forgot, or forgave a transgression.

I have a slight tendency to ramble on a bit, so you'll have to keep an eye on me for that. Back to my earliest memory. Mother had told me that on the night I was born it was snowing. She said I was many weeks past my due date and she was in a world of pain and suffering. She was all bloated and swollen and was feeling awful. My sister was only eighteen months old, so life was difficult. She stoically ploughed on as was the lot of women in London in 1963 (if you've ever watched *Call the Midwife* on telly, you can almost picture the scene). Well, she just kept going until she collapsed whereupon my Dad called the cavalry and she was rushed into hospital by ambulance, or *under lights* as she called it (I credit her for my flair for drama). I was dragged into the world not breathing, blue-black in colour, with my skin peeling off. According to Mother it was a terrible business and she just knew I'd be nothing but trouble. Right from the get-go I was a bloody nuisance. So, "What does that have to do with the hairy therapist?" you ask, well...

He set up a video camera to tape our session, which was meant to reassure me that no funny business would take place whilst I was under hypnosis. The thought had never occurred to me until he said that by the way. Gulp! Anyhow it all seemed straight forward enough. I would lie back in a big recliner chair, covered by a blanket to preserve my modesty. He would talk me through the session and I could communicate via hand signals all the way through. He assured me I had complete control over the process. Well, as it turns out, that wasn't quite how it went down. He went through the finger signals to communicate yes, no, stop and so on (no middle fingers were used in this demonstration). He would talk and I would reveal the inner most secrets of my convoluted mind. He would set me on the right path immediately after waking me up, fully alert and feeling refreshed.

Woo-woo (I mean peaceful, meditative) music playing quietly in the background, relaxing oils burning on the burner, he sat on his chair next to the giant recliner I was tucked into and I closed my eyes. He tapped my hand and we went through the signals again to be sure I was still ok. I indicated that I was and we were off! I was instructed to imagine myself as a small white pebble. I did mention I was there for a weight issue, didn't I? I think I snorted at that point and was sharply admonished to still my mind and concentrate on his voice. Duly chastened, I obediently raised my index finger to indicate I understood and would behave and off we went again. The small white pebble (me) was dropped into the water. "Water, what water?" Tap, tap, tap went the hairy finger and once again I subsided, waved "Sorry" with my index finger and tried to follow him. But come on, this is weird shit! I was questioning everything, my mind was racing a mile a minute, I was convinced this was a load of crock and I was as far from relaxed as a deer caught in the crosshairs of a loaded gun. Then he said, "Where are you?"

I don't even know how to explain what happened to me next. Suddenly I was being squeezed from all sides, it was pitch dark, hot, claustrophobic and unbearable. I started to panic, my heart beating furiously and the infernal squeezing from all sides was relentless. In the distance I could hear his voice telling me I was quite safe, that I was all right. Then again that same question, "Where are you?" Then suddenly, there was a bright light and so much noise. People with masks and gowns on were shouting and there was blood everywhere. I realized with absolute shocking clarity, that I had just been born! I told you this was weird shit.

Completely stunned I lay mute and still. Again, I heard that voice, but this time he said, "What do you need?" I heard myself reply, "I need someone to hold me." I have never experienced a longing to be held as exquisitely, painfully and completely primal as I did in that moment. That need consumed me like a wildfire and became all that I could think about. But no one held me. I was smacked across my bottom and then put into a box and the lid was closed. I could see outside my incubator (Mother had told me about that... I stayed in it for three weeks I believe). Everyone was running around; they were trying to save Mother's life.

As I lay there in that box, the need to be held slowly drained from my body to be replaced with an absolute knowing that I was completely on my own and I had better get used to it or leave now. "When do they hold you?" asked the voice, that by now seemed so far removed from where I was lying in total abject misery, willing myself to die, that I almost didn't hear it. Tap, tap, tap went the finger and again, but more urgently this time, "When do they hold you?"

"When they feed me," I heard myself whisper, as the world went black and I became invisible.

I was brought back to reality by a furious tapping on my hand and some urgent sounding entreaties by the hairy therapist who looked rather shaken himself. I had turned completely upside down in the recliner chair and whilst I struggled to rearrange myself, he sat in his chair blinking like a crazed owl. I can't recall how we ended the session, but I left there in a daze that lasted for over two decades. I felt inexorably changed, but in a way that I could not identify with, nor understand. That day changed the trajectory of my life and sent me on a voyage of discovery that has involved some really weird shit. I'd like to share some bits and pieces of that voyage with you if you'd like to hear about it. Perhaps some of the weird shit I learned along the way will resonate with you and will help you to know yourself a little better. Because that was the overriding question in my mind after being birthed again at the age of thirty-something by a hairy-as-fuck midwife, "Who am I?" and "Why am I here?"

Life Lessons:

- Sometimes you need to get right out of your comfort zone to find the answers (or at least the beginning of the road toward finding the answers)
- You need to surrender control if you want to learn your truth
- You may need to experience some weird shit to survive this life
- Food equals comfort
- Hairy men are indeed scary!

Chapter 2

The childhood conundrum

After my dramatic entrance into the world, I apparently became a very angry infant. I screamed night and day for a full ten months. My sister apparently took one look at me and told our Mother, "I don't like it, take it away again." I think this opinion was shared by all who suffered through my horrendous, unrelenting, screaming fits. One night (and I will come back to this later in my journey), Mother reached the end of her tether. She would tell anyone who would listen, (including many iterations of the same sentiment to me as an adult), that I was a *dreadful baby*. One night she had had enough of me. She dropped me head-first into my cot, tossed in a bottle of milk and told me to, "Just bloody get on with it then, I've had enough of you!" She walked out, shut the door and that was that. At that point I stopped crying and I didn't start again until fifty years later.

I'm certain Mother thought she had finally gotten through to me and congratulated herself on a sterling parenting move. I must be honest here and say I totally empathise with her. It can't be fun being saddled with a full time screaming infant and a two-year-old. Also did I mention Mother was forty-three when I was born? I do, however, remain steadfastly opposed to the idea that dropping your baby on its head is a means of teaching it a lesson. I am pleased to say I never once resorted to that whilst raising my own daughters.

I retreated into myself, once again fully certain that I was in this on my own, but this time shielding an anger that was so powerful, it almost evaporated me. It's tough being an infant who is dependent on others for, well, literally everything, but who has declared in her little ten-month-old mind and heart the infant equivalent of, "Well fuck you too! Okay, I'll keep quiet. I'll take care of myself. I won't take anything from you, I don't need you either." Naturally this is impossible to do and the resulting build-up of resentment, frustration and anger, wholly underpinned by a soul level sadness, confounded by the inability to speak up, created a seething mass of repressed feelings. Of course, at the time I didn't understand any of this and simply became a mute, confused little child. I hid behind a mask of platitude. I did what was expected of me and went quietly back into my box immediately after. I became an invisible child, as close to not being there as I could achieve while still breathing.

Somewhere inside of me the rage raged on. I wet my bed until I was ten years old. That earned me the title every morning of *filthy little pig*. It's a great way to start your day especially after you've been kneeling on the floor all night huffing and puffing and blowing until you are dizzy, trying to dry the damning wet patch. Mother was convinced I did it just to vex her and to make her life a living hell. I suppose, if I'm being fair, it did add a substantial burden to her day. I grew up in a different world from the one we live in today. There were no therapists or supports available to her; and let's not forget that she was also governed by *them*, and any failing of mine, reflected poorly on her in *their* eyes. Neither of us realised we were caught in this awful dance between her and me and *them*. I will explain more about *them* later on I promise. If you're a bit confused right now, then great, you're right where I was at growing up.

At the age of four, I started school. That's quite usual for English children. A whole new realm of confusion opened before me like a gaping chasm, just waiting for me to stumble into it. I don't know how it happened, but I just seemed to spend my entire childhood feeling confused, never knowing where I needed to be, or what was going on. If, by some miracle, I did arrive in the right place, then I didn't know why I was there in the first place. It was as though everyone else had been fully briefed on life, whilst I had slept through the whole thing. I was wary of the other children, terrified of the teachers and confused by the loud bell that resulted in mass movement of people like ants in a colony. I trusted no one, myself least of all. I remember I had a coat peg at my school with a picture of a Red Robin on it. I was told it was my special place. There was many a time when four-year-old me was found hiding behind my coat at my special place.

There was an innate rhythm to life at school, but I had no idea how to do the dance. My dance classes in life had been more primal and survival based. I learned the *How to be Seen and Not Heard Tango*, the *Duck and Dive Jive*, the *Don't you Embarrass me Cha-cha*, and my personal favourite, the *I'll Belt you if you Cross me Waltz*. I do think however, it was the *Speak Only When Spoken to Salsa* that really gummed up my poor little brain. Everything in me screamed out to ask for direction and instruction (some people call this help, others call it parenting), but my experiences in life had taught me that no one was there to help me. My job was to remain invisible and not cause trouble. I had no clue how to proceed and so I remained a bed wetting, nervous wreck, the brunt of class ridicule, with a confused look on my face… Mother called this my *gormless face*.

At the age of seven, we emigrated to South Africa. Naturally I didn't have a clue what that meant, but I do remember one evening everyone was dressed in their Sunday best, we had suitcases and we were driven somewhere in a taxi. It was most confusing. I remember being dragged by my hand along a corridor with so many strange people. Suddenly, as if by magic we were in a new place. It was crowded and narrow and there were rows and rows of strange people in seats all staring at us. We were on a plane, in case that's not clear. There had been some confusion with the booking and we only had three seats side by side. Naturally as the undesirable family member, I was dispatched to sit between two nuns who promised to watch me and make sure I didn't cause a problem. As I sit here writing, I can see it vividly in my mind. I can smell the plane, feel the prickly maroon fabric of the seat beneath my legs as I sat there all dressed up in my best pink crimplene dress with the brown lace on the collar and I want to cry. My chest feels tight and I don't want to breathe in case I get into trouble. I was terrified and to this day, I have an utter aversion to nuns in habit which is ridiculous of course as I am certain they were incredibly kind to me, although I cannot recall.

Resolving childhood trauma is like peeling an onion, let me assure you the layers of the onion are endless. Long after you think you've dealt with the onion, fried the bloody thing even, or tossed it out altogether, another little bit surfaces for you to look at and cry over. Regardless, fast forward to a new school in a new country with a new language, new customs and rituals. How do you think I did? Well, I made a massive three-sixty turnaround and became the star of the school, most popular girl, an academic force to be reckoned with and an all-round exemplary student, admired by all who encountered me...NOT!

Life Lessons:

- Be seen and not heard
- Speak only when spoken to
- Life sucks
- Red Robins are safe
- Nuns are scary

Chapter 3

The thespian conundrum

One thing I did discover when I arrived in the South African schooling system, is that I was way ahead of the curve when it came to reading skills. Whilst my contemporaries at aged seven mastered the art of *See Spot Run* and the machinations of *Janet and John,* I was lost in the world of Enid Blyton. It stands to reason that books became my refuge, my safe place, my way to explore and have adventures. I developed my character under cover of silence and secrecy. *They* never knew what I read and I discovered I could have a tremendous time inside the pages of a book in relative safety. I just had to remember to do my chores, not cause trouble and keep my joy invisible. If I managed that correctly, then Mother never knew either and I was home free. In fact, that is exactly what I did and so when I credit myself with anything resembling a normal childhood, I confess it was all from within the pages of books and is mostly fictional. I developed a great imagination and I thrived in my imaginary world. There, I was protected, fully informed and was in fact, quite clever. It was me who solved the mysteries and acted as the hero of the piece, rescuing those less fortunate. I lived to read.

When I was eight, I took part in a school play. I recall having to enter stage right carrying a book and my great line was, "Is the French for book Li or La?" (It is of course *livre*). I don't remember anything else about the play, what it was called, or what it was about. I was positively bursting with excitement. At last I was going to be visible. I was feeling brave as a result of my reading adventures and I was determined that this play would be the vehicle that would change my life forever. My parents would be proud of me and would tell everyone about their talented child. On the afternoon of the play, I donned my new red patent leather shoes. They were the most incredible thing I had ever owned and I did everything I could to ensure they were not taken away from me. Those shoes made me feel like Dorothy, from the *Wizard of Oz;* they made a wondrous staccato clipping sound when I walked. Anyway, I waited in the wings with bated breath and right on cue I stepped out onto the stage.

"Walk properly!" Mother had said. "Don't embarrass me!" I had this. I had prepared so well for this. I knew my line; I was ready to be seen. I placed the heel of my shiny red shoe on the newly polished stage and I went into a skid. Arms and legs akimbo, the book went flying and I slid into one of the principle actors taking her legs out from under her. We both lay in a tangle of limbs, horrified and embarrassed. The audience loved it and applause broke out from all corners of the auditorium. I looked up blinking like a startled owl. Stunned by their response, I gathered myself, took a calming breath and delivered my line with the aplomb of a seasoned Shakespearian thespian. This resulted in even more laughter from the audience. I scrambled up, whispered "Sorry," to the other actor, who by now was crying and tottered off carefully back to the wings, kind of like Bambi on Ice. That was the last time Mother ever set foot inside of a school building; and I never saw my red shoes again.

Fast forward to ten-years-old and I have an English teacher who tells me I have enormous potential. I learned to hate the word potential. It meant (and did for most of my life) that someone had an expectation of me that I wouldn't fully understand and would therefore disappoint at. That bloody word has caused me to become paralysed and stuck in so many situations I could have easily resolved. Anyway, there I was being accused of having potential. "I'd like you to audition for the school play," she said. "I think it will be really good for your confidence." "Are you friggin' kidding me!!!!!" I want to scream, but I've been taught not to push back and to accept every piece of shit that life throws at me without complaint. So, I smiled and said, "Wow, that's so exciting. Thank you so much, I can't wait." No matter how badly I tried to do at the audition, the potential won the day and I landed a speaking role.

Rehearsals were during school time, so I didn't have to invoke the wrath of *them*, by upsetting the routines of the household. It didn't cost anything, my teacher agreed to subsidize my costume when I told her my parents would never agree to spend money on something so frivolous. I would be barefoot, so I wouldn't be skating on the stage. Oh boy. This could happen. I made the fatal error of allowing myself to get excited. I prepared, I worked hard, I was especially diligent at home and didn't annoy anyone. I had an incredible costume. A Japanese kimono made from a beautiful pink and black silky material that transported me to another world, it was so grand. We were three days away from dress rehearsal when I hit a snag. The show would be at night which meant I would need to be taken to school and collected again. That was all outside of the routine of the household and would be construed as a transgression of the highest order. I told my teacher I could no longer be in the play. She laughed and said, "Don't be so silly. Would you like me to talk to your Mother?" Well, now I knew that I was done for. *They* would find out what I had been doing and all hell would break loose. Having the school phone Mother was tantamount to treason. How do you, as a muted child, explain this to a kind, but ignorant teacher. She was incredible and made a most reasonable case on my behalf. She even offered to drive me there and back herself. Mother was all charm and sweetness and agreed that of course I could be in the play. Like a fool, I was overjoyed.

The next afternoon however, Mother told me I had to go to the doctors. I suffered terribly from sore throats my whole childhood. Mother decided that it needed to be seen to immediately. Off to the doctor's office I was dragged and arrangements were made for me to have my tonsils removed… on the day of the play. The smug expression on her face is something that will live with me forever as she said, "Did you think you'd get to embarrass me again? I don't think so." I had to go to school and tell my teacher that I really couldn't be in the play. I was gutted. She was furious, but somehow, I don't think it was me she was angry at. I imagined it was because she had one day to rehearse an understudy, refit a costume and all the other production problems my pulling out would cause her. She was incredibly kind to me and said I would be allowed to attend the dress rehearsal. No one was supposed to watch a dress rehearsal and the gesture was designed to make me feel better I suppose. I allowed myself a few discreet, quiet tears that afternoon as I watched Arlene!!! Parading around in my kimono, saying my lines. I so badly wanted her to trip and fall, but she was perfect. The play was ready. I was off to hospital. The nurses were nuns. I almost bled to death as a result of a post-operative complication.

Life lessons:

- Revenge is Mother's and *they* always win in the end
- Nuns ARE scary
- One should never get too hopeful or optimistic
- Sometimes even a great teacher can't save you, although it's incredible when they try - Miss Burgess, I know what you tried to do. Thank you.

Chapter 4

The religious conundrum

I ended up being a halfway decent student. Throughout my entire primary school experience, I was only ever sent to the headmaster's office once. He opened the door, took one look at me and said, "No, this must be a mistake! Go back to class my dear." I managed to forge a few tentative relationships, nothing near friendship, but they allowed me inclusion on the periphery of certain activities and situations. For the most part however, I was the outsider of the school. The adults all saw my mysterious *potential*, although it remained elusive in my sight; the children, not so much. I guess in that age group life is all about quid pro quo. Kids swapped stories about holidays (I never went on one); they exchanged goodies from their lunchboxes (I wasn't allowed to eat outside of the house); they arranged playdates (I wasn't allowed to go anywhere after school, except home to my room); they invited each other to their birthday parties (I never had one); they swapped clothes (you're kidding right!); they played sport (that would have been outside of school hours so, just no!). I can see looking back, why I was a bit of an enigma to them.

I recall one evening when I was eleven, we had all piled into the car after dinner and drove to the corner café to buy chocolate bars. Chocolate bars were the equivalent of good boy chocolate drops in our life. If we got through a whole week without anyone having to be given a good hiding, or anyone upsetting Mother, we were taken to buy a chocolate bar. I was feeling strange. My head hurt and my skin was all prickly. My eyes ached so badly and I was shivering. I really didn't want to say anything and spoil the treat, but I think I may have groaned out loud. Mother's head snapped round and she glared at me. "What's wrong with you?" she growled. Cornered and feeling awful, I mumbled, "I'm really sorry, but I don't feel well." My sister set up a ruckus, my Dad sighed, Mother started ranting and raving. The car was turned around and we went back home. I was given a hiding for spoiling the whole family's outing. I was sent to bed. Turned out I had the measles. When the doctor came the following Monday and pronounced thus, I was given black cherries and lemonade to drink as a treat. I still hate black cherries and lemonade.

Weird Shit!

You might be wondering why my sister set up a ruckus in the last story. Well, it was probably because the poor girl had to suffer through having a car sick, mute little sister. Every time we went anywhere in the car, I ended up feeling dizzy and car sick. I knew better than to say anything and invoke the wrath of *them,* so I would jiggle my foot furiously and pretend I was alright. I would visit the characters in my current book in my mind and pretend I wasn't even in the car. Well it didn't always work and I had an alarming habit of vomiting all over my sister. It's no wonder she hated me growing up! So many family photographs with my sister wearing the emergency beach wear that was kept in the back of the car. So much evidence of my shame.

High school was another matter entirely. Perhaps the hormones gave me courage. I met some incredible girls and forged brilliant friendships. One of those girls is still a best friend today. High school was pure Nirvana to me. I played sport – tennis, swimming and netball (there were additional busses to accommodate the lateness so I could sort myself out); I played musical instruments, violin for one term until my teacher begged me to stop for the sake of her hearing; clarinet for about the same time and stopped for the same reason; then finally the recorder, which the school gave me free. That's right, I played the recorder in the high school orchestra and what of it! I was the choir leader too and I had a badge to prove it. My friends got me involved in horse riding. I could spend weekends at their homes after a fair amount of political debate and some seriously great tap-dancing manoeuvres on my part. Those times spent riding and hanging out with the horses gave me some of my happiest memories. Weekends away were oases in the desert that was my home life. I joined a church youth movement with my best friend where I sang in the church choir, often solo. There were so many highlights that it became easier to haze over the other stuff. Finally, I was gaining some visibility.

Unfortunately, *they* remained in control of Mother and terrorised her endlessly, which she in turn passed on to me. For some reason *they* didn't bother with my sister. When I turned sixteen, Mother seemed to be gripped by a fear and certainty that I was going to become some sort of scarlet woman who would heap shame and ridicule upon our house. This is still a little strange to me because she made no effort at all to educate me in the ways of the world, on what becoming a woman was all about, how to behave around boys or what to expect from my body. Thank heavens for friends, although they aren't always the best sources of information having their own agendas to deal with. I frequently found myself falling foul of her unreasonable fears.

I loved Friday evenings as I could go to the Apostolic Church's youth guild. It was a big stretch for Mother, but as my Dad said, "It's church for goodness sake, what could possibly happen to her there?" I'll always be grateful he did not allude to what I might do, but instead to what might befall me. He believed in my innocence. The Pastor had three gorgeous young sons who were breathtakingly handsome. One of them had a friend staying over, and they all had big 1300cc Kawasaki motorbikes. The friend was good looking, mysterious, had a beard, was out of school and did I mention the motorbike! He was dangerous on the Richter scale. My darling friend, who had no problem at all with any level of maleness, managed to persuade them to take us on the back of their motorbikes to an ice cream hut on the beach front. I figured it was 8pm and I should be able to hit my curfew of 10pm so I'd be alright. No one ever needed to know. I allowed myself to be pinioned and enjoyed a thrilling ride. The ice cream stop went on way past 10pm and I knew I was in for a world of pain, but I had no chance of convincing the others that they should cut their evening short, just because Mother was a tyrant. So, I kept on smiling and laughing, all the while building up the dreaded fear on the inside. At 11pm I was dropped at home and Mother met me at the door with a slap that knocked me off my feet. I was called a filthy slut. I tried to explain that I had wanted to come home, but… Slap!!! "You don't eat ice cream at eleven o'clock at night!" Long, miserable episode cut short, I was banned from seeing my friend, from going to youth guild and from anything outside of the house for the rest of time, with the obvious and grudging exception of school. My Dad stood silently by while this tirade went on and somehow, I felt a solidarity with him. He too, had learned to be invisible.

It took a long time for the dust to settle, but eventually it did. I was once again allowed to go to church services, if not youth. I was dropped at the appropriate time and collected one minute after service was due to have finished. I feel I need to be honest here and tell you that I had not one ounce of religious conviction. I went purely for the sense of belonging to a community. It was a place where I was encouraged and even celebrated; and I got to sing. I spoke to the Pastor about what was going on, since he wanted to know why I had dropped out of youth. I was part of their youth choir and he wanted me to come back. He wanted to talk to my parents. All I could think about was if getting a teacher to advocate for me got my tonsils removed (I will literally cut your throat to stop you from speaking – dramatic interpretation!!), I dreaded to imagine what getting a Pastor to talk to them might incite. The correct action in this circumstance, advised the good Pastor, was that I was to be baptised. Once I was a certified child of God my parents would be ok with me going back to youth. I heard myself say, "I would love to be baptised! Thank you for asking me." I still struggle to say no. Besides, I did enjoy the idea of being part of a group, of being accepted and of getting into God's good graces. He seemed to have been conspicuous by His absence thus far, so perhaps it wouldn't hurt to dig in a bit into His territory.

I approached my Dad about the subject of a baptism and he was supportive. It was almost as if he liked the idea of us having something special between us. He came to church to watch me do my dunk and save bit and he even bought me a book called *Great People of the Bible and How They Lived*. I never read it though because he inscribed it to me with a wish that I would find a *better way of being*. The Pastor said he was disappointed that I didn't come out of the water speaking in tongues. Yet again, someone who saw my potential was disappointed because I, once again, had missed the brief. Oh well. At least I could go and sing in the youth choir again which was really all I had wanted out of the whole affair in the first place. One of my greatest joys was singing Amazing Grace or How Great Thou Art and watching the emotion on the faces of the congregation as they seemed to soar with the notes I arched into the rafters. They perhaps didn't see me, Janice, but they couldn't deny my presence and I felt powerful as I connected with them through the music.

At sixteen, I had gone to spend the weekend at a friend's home. Her church was holding a disco for the youth. Imagine! I was going to a disco, without adult supervision. Ok, I was dressed like something out of *Anne of Green Gables* and I had no idea how to dance; and after the motorbike episode I was scared stupid to be near anything resembling a boy, but I had enough girl power around me to pull me through. And of course, we shouldn't forget about those courageous hormones. There's only so much one can do with a pot-on-head home brew haircut, but I could borrow clothes and even wear makeup. Off we went and I still don't know if it was more thrilling or terrifying. Once again, I'd missed the brief. Everyone was drinking and swaying to the music, gripping tightly onto one another, or just laughing and chatting, but I was completely overwhelmed. I knew that within the walls of that darkened place lay the beginnings of my ruin. I knew that *they* would know I was there and that nothing good could come of my being present. Once again though, I can't do anything to save myself and so I just shrink into a corner and pull down my invisibility shield. One of the boys came over and tried to chat to me. I almost threw up I was so scared. He seemed to take my mute responses as encouragement and moved himself in between my knees. He slipped his hand up inside my skirt and did unmentionable things with his fingers. I was utterly paralysed with fear until he tried to kiss me. He stank of beer. I squealed "No!" shoved him away and ran outside to the sound of his drunken laughter. Many hours later my friend came and found me. She had had a wonderful evening as was evidenced by the redness of her chin and the atomic glow of her eyes. I never said a word. We were collected by her father who pronounced himself satisfied that we were neither drunk nor disorderly and we were told to get to bed and admonished not to be late for church in the morning. I fell asleep listening to my friend prattling on about how amazing it was kissing boys and how she couldn't wait to have sex someday.

The following Monday Mother came to collect my sister and I from school. As we arrived home, I was treated to a resounding smack across the side of my face. A litany of filthy language and accusations were levied at me. Apparently, the randy lothario had gone and spread it around school what a great lay I was and how I was so easy. If the guys wanted a good time to seek out 0800-JAN-CAN. I could make no defence, he had touched me there and I hadn't stopped him, even though it was fear that had made me freeze. Perhaps I deserved all of this. Maybe she was right and I was a filthy slut. I simply had to endure while I was lectured about the shame and disgrace and ... oh God it just went on and on including how I had tarnished my sister's sterling reputation. "But we won't tell your Father!" Well that surprised me. My Dad was always loving and for the most part fair. He failed however, to protect me from Mother (it took me a lot of weird shit sessions to be able to say that); and if it was a choice between throwing me under the bus or keeping the peace with Mother, he always went her way. I wasn't sure what I thought he could have done for me in that situation, but I knew that by being denied any possibility of his support, I was being punished in the most extreme way. I believe she was punishing him too for supporting me in the great baptism betrayal.

One weekend when I was staying at my friend's house, we again went to her church's youth guild. They were showing a movie that her parents decided we needed to see. It was called The Rapture and it remains to this day one of the most shocking things I have ever seen. I think the intention was to convince young Christian children that life was finite and the consequences for not living 'right' were dire. I already knew all about the consequences of not living right so I wasn't too worried. I sat in that dark church a young, impressionable teen, developmentally unable to distinguish anything in context with reality, watching those two terrifying old film reels. People finding themselves abandoned by their loved ones, their friends, colleagues and community, with panicked news readers breathlessly reporting on the mystery of so many people simply vanishing in the space of a moment, and the ensuing chaos and fear. This was followed up by a drive to gather up all the remaining people and mark them with the 666-brand identifying them as loyal followers of the state. Those who held on to their Christian principles and refused the mark, were put to death.

This gruesome and terrifying offering was then followed by a call to the alter, for us children to dedicate our lives to the Lord to ensure that we would not be left behind when the time came.

I already knew I was an undesirable, *they* had made that quite clear. For me, the thought of being undesirable even to God in heaven seemed a very real possibility. In the company of my friend and every other child there we sold our souls to fear and insecurity. I went through the motions, but I was devastated having finally been shown proof from someone other than Mother, that I had no value whatsoever. On that night I dedicated myself, not to God, but to becoming a walking service industry simply to justify my existence. I would create value for myself by becoming useful. I promised to do whatever I was told or asked to do just to be allowed to exist and I shut myself down completely. That night, thanks to what I now consider an act of spiritual terrorism by the church, who were supposed to guide and lead us, I became a walking service industry, less human, more commodity.

One way or another I managed to get through school in relatively good form. In my final year I was awarded the *Service to the School* prize at prizegiving and was presented with a little white leather King James bible. I was rather pleased with that because it seemed proof that my choice to be of service was the right one. I wrote my last exam on a Thursday and the following Monday I started working at a bank. One of the good Pastors' sons had recommended me for a position as a junior clerk. The branch manager was full-on God squad and because I came in baptised and church endorsed, I could do no wrong. Prayer meetings in the mornings with entreaties to God on High to keep us honest in our accounting were a bit awkward, but by then I'd done more than a few drama classes, had hidden myself successfully in plain sight all of my life and I pulled it off from behind my mask. I still hadn't seen much evidence of God showing up in my life, but I wasn't averse to using His good name to help myself out.

Life Lessons:

- There is no God
- Boys suck
- I can manipulate people into thinking I'm a good person
- I'll never get to Heaven
- Music and singing are where all the joy in the world is hidden

Chapter 5

The Jewish conundrum

I joined a volleyball team with one of my work mates who was desperate for someone to be worse at volleyball than she, even if only for one night until I learned to play properly. The volleyball coach spoke so quietly that I couldn't hear a word he said. I watched him mime the movements of dig, set, spike and I watched the other players until I had it down pat. Didn't help that he had a full-face beard and his mumbling words were lost in that great hairiness. Turns out I'm not that great at jumping and I was forced to have extra attention to improve that skill. By the time I'd learned to hop about successfully we were dating and then somehow, I had managed to get myself engaged to a Jewish doctor. Mother was over the moon and for a brief period she suspended her venomous dance routine. I spoke to the good Pastor about the Jewish business since apparently, I was required to convert to Judaism. It appears there was nowhere I could go in life where I was acceptable as is. The good Pastor hugged me and said, "It doesn't matter where you are my dear child, as long as you let your light shine bright." I had a light. I was a light? Who knew!

As fiancés tend to do, we ended up having sex and I knew that I would have to marry this man since I was now officially ruined and spoiled. Mother's words rang ever present in my head, "Who would want someone like you? You'll be lucky to find anyone who will put up with you. No self-respecting man will marry a slut who's been with other men." It was no longer 1922, but I had been schooled hard and I knew I had crossed a line of respectability and my fate was sealed. The guilt was giving me hives. He seemed to be a very nice man though and it was exciting to try out adulthood with him. I counted my blessings and feeling grateful that, for whatever reason, someone wanted to be with me, I accepted his proposal. I had such high hopes for marriage. I dreamed of finally being visible, of having someone in life who would always be pleased to see me and who would prioritise my well-being in line with his, instead of always taking the path of least resistance to keep the peace. I had no experience of love and such grandiose notions were not for the likes of people like me so I didn't worry myself unduly on that score. In retrospect I was far too young and naïve to be marrying anyone, but I had no real concept of me having a choice in the matter. In my experience life happened to you and you didn't push back or rock the boat for fear of retribution. So, off to the alter it would be, except in this case it was under the chuppah.

Since I was required to become someone other than who I was in order to be with him, I attended conversion classes and learned to adopt yet another mask. We hit a snag when my Jewish mother-in-law, true to tradition, created merry hell about my inherent lack of Jewishness. It didn't seem to matter that I was already bending over backwards to meet the requirements and was turning my back on my own way of life, traditions and beliefs. In all honesty there wasn't much that bothered me besides Christmas. She took every opportunity to let me know that as far as she was concerned, I was a huge disappointment. She went too far one day when she said to me, "You will marry my son over my dead body!" Well that was it. The die was cast, I would marry this man if it was the last thing I did. That little ten-month-old baby inside of me found her voice. In a newly adult voice she declared, "You just watch me!" In case you're wondering, that's scared twenty-year-old for "Well fuck you too!" I couldn't bear to have another dominating maternal figure hating my every move and my very existence. At least this one didn't come with an accompanying *them,* so I started to fight back.

Fiancé's sage advice was to not take it personally. With the wisdom of the passing years, I do realise he was right. If I had just realised this was her custom, her way of dealing with life, and in fact, it had very little to do with me personally, we would have been just fine. But, twenty years of not being good enough was starting to rumble inside of me and I was struggling to keep *me* suppressed. It felt very personal to me and I quickly became sick and tired of being told I wasn't good enough for her son, especially when her son never took my part or defended me in any way. Battle lines were drawn and it took many years before we called a truce. Fiancé became yet another significant male figure in my life who would always acquiesce to the Mother. I was once again left feeling abandoned, on my own in life, confused and not quite understanding the brief. I was officially converted to Judaism on a Friday – I read the wrong passage to the congregation from my lofty place on the bimah, but as I said to the Rabbi, no one was paying attention anyway so what did it really matter. He laughed and said, "You're going to fit right it." I turned twenty-one on the Saturday – fiancé forgot it was my birthday. We were married on Sunday – and that was the end of Solomon Grundy.

I discovered I was claustrophobic on my honeymoon. We had gone climbing in a series of caves and at one point I became wedged in a very narrow part and had a panic attack. To the annoyance of all the other intrepid climbers, I had to be hauled feet first out of the cave's narrow passage. I was left alone in an enormous dark cave to find my own way back to the entrance whilst Husband and the others, continued their experience. That night when he climbed on top of me, I had another panic attack. I fought like a lion and threw the poor, startled sod onto the floor. I jumped up clutching the sheet and with wild eyes, I screamed at him, "You left me alone in the fucking cave on our honeymoon!!!!" I felt completely alone, abandoned, unworthy of his protection or his priority. Any illusions I had of feeling safe in this relationship faded away and I realised that if this marriage was to survive, I would have to stay buried and work out how to fit in without attracting too much attention. I would work out the dance steps for marriage and I would continue to stay invisible. I would not be able to grow into my elusive potential. I've heard that light will always find a way and in the back of my mind I could hear the good Pastor saying, "Just let your light shine bright." That little epiphany was however, quickly quashed and sent back to the shadows where it belonged.

I adopted the mask of happy wife and played my part for all I was worth. My internal sadness grew a little more each day. My disappointment grew exponentially. I was well and truly stuck, but as Mother frequently told me, "You made your bed my girl, you damned well lie in it." We had some very good times and it wasn't all bad, but we never really seemed to talk. I felt as though we were going through the motions of life without actually engaging with it. If I didn't extend my thinking past the end of the nose on my face, I managed just fine.

One incredible thing Husband did do for me, was to buy me my first horse. My old school friend had married into a racing family and they had an ex racehorse that she wanted to send to me. He was just standing in the bush not being ridden and she knew him to be an incredible horse. Well people like us (that's another Mother-gem letting me know that I had no station in life and shouldn't expect anything good because I didn't deserve it), just didn't own ex racehorses, but by some glorious miracle it turned out… we did!

The excitement on the day the horse carrier arrived from out of town was palpable. I will never forget that day for so many reasons. Primarily it was a day of huge disappointment, but also the day I learned to have faith, a completely alien concept to me. Looking back, it was also a day filled with irony. I tore down to the stables at the allotted time and waited with bated breath as my horse was backed out of the trailer. He was a very tall, rail thin chestnut, with a short scrubby tail; his hooves were overgrown and cracked and his coat was long and scruffy. He was clearly exhausted from the journey and he stood with his head down looking utterly forlorn. This was no racehorse. Of course, I patted him and said hello, but the disappointment was oozing out of every pore. That poor horse, what a shocking way I greeted his arrival. Not with love and joy and gratitude, but with disappointment. The stable manager squinted at him, then at my face and he came over to me and said, "Can you trust me and have faith that this is a good thing happening here?" Well, by now you get that I'm not big on trust and have no experience with faith at all, but options were few and far between so I nodded, not trusting my quavering voice to speak. He said I should stay away from the stables and he would phone me when I could come and see the horse again. I went home, thanked Husband profusely for buying me a horse and went on with the business of working and living.

By this stage I was working in a laboratory as a medical technician. I gave up banking when the chief sub accountant couldn't keep his hands to himself and it became too awkward for me to work with him. He was a manager (big) and I was eighteen and naïve (small). So, instead of reporting his disgusting ass, I just left and scuttled off into the night. I met a friend on the bus on my way home. I was wondering how I would explain to Mother that I'd left my job and didn't have any idea what I was going to do or how I would pay my rent that month. The friend told me they were looking for lab technicians at the Blood Bank where she worked. She arranged an interview for me the next day. I got the job and voila, I was training to be a medical technologist. I loved my time in the laboratories, testing donor blood to ensure it was safe for patient use; running compatibility tests between donor and patient; all manner of exciting things that put me on the periphery of the medical world. Okay, now I did warn you that I tend to ramble, so, back to married life and the stables.

It was three months before the call came in from the stable manager. I went to the yard and he greeted me looking quite pleased with himself. "Go and see your boy," he said, "he's in that barn over there." I entered the barn and strolled through greeting all the inquisitive heads that popped over doors to see who was there. I didn't see my boy and figured the manager had made a mistake about where he was standing. I was about to leave when from the last stable at the end, appeared the wide rounded neck and giant head of the most magnificent animal I had ever seen in my life. Veins stood out on his sleek neck and his coat looked like it was made of spun copper. He stood with his head high, ears pricked and looked right at me. I remember my breath catching in my throat as I stood rooted to the spot. I felt a little like Icarus looking too closely at the sun (alright that's a terrible and inaccurate analogy, but it makes the point quite dramatically). Now that's what I had expected a racehorse to look like! I backed out of the barn resisting the urge to bow before the magnificent horse. I wondered who was lucky enough to own such an incredible beast. I walked back to the manager who was busy with a client. He grinned when I shrugged to indicate no luck finding my horse. He waved a stable lad over to go and bring my horse out. I busied myself daydreaming while I waited. Hearing hooves clopping on the cobbles, I turned around and walking towards me was the magnificent chestnut horse from the end stable. Once again, my breath caught in my chest as I gazed in awe at the incredible beast. I still didn't get it. The manager was by now rolling with laughter. "That's your horse, you idiot!" he managed to wheeze out between giant snorts of laughter. Thus, began my first official love affair.

Life Lessons:

- Disappointment is a way of life
- Fighting back is futile
- I'll never be good enough
- No one has my back
- Horses bring you joy

Chapter 6

The parenting conundrum

Life bumbled along at a satisfactory pace. Between work, riding, running a home and maintaining a relationship we moved along from A to B on a relatively even keel. My happiest hours were spent riding, or just sitting in my horses feed-trough with his big, beautiful head resting in my lap, breathing him in and revelling in the pure energy of him. I competed in a few show jumping events, rode the odd cross country and even attempted a little dressage. Nothing thrilled me quite as much as the feeling of complete freedom as we rode out on the farm with the sun in our faces and the wind at our backs (Ok, now I'm starting to sound like an Irish proverb).

I have no recollection of how we got there (I'm still largely confounded by life and its complicated requirements), but at some point, we arrived at the next logical step in our relationship and I was pregnant. Did I think about the implications of having a child? Did I have a parenting plan? A birthing plan? A friggin' clue…? No. I rode my horse until two weeks before my baby was born simply because it never occurred to me not to. I only stopped because I fell off in the forest one day and was too big and bulky to get back on and had to walk all the way back to the yard. If you are familiar with the concept of guardian angels, then it is reasonable to suppose that mine were probably taking out restraining orders against me at that point.

Don't get me wrong, I was excited to be having a baby. I'd decorated a nursery, knitted a baby blanket, taken my vitamins, seen my doctor and apart from thinking I would be the first person to die of heartburn and having all-day sickness for five months, I had loved being pregnant. Those sacred moments when it's just you and the baby moving inside of you. It must be the most selfish feeling, like being privy to the greatest secret in the world. I was winging it on pure instinct at this point because I didn't know any better. I can't remember much us-ness through the experience, but I know I loved it all.

Labour was a huge shock! Somewhere along the way, I had forgotten the life lesson of not getting too optimistic. I had cramp in both my legs from being in stirrups for hours and the assault on my senses was overwhelming as the epidural wore off when it came time to push. My body is not designed for bringing new life into the world. I had laboured for fourteen hours, shielded for a blissful eight of them by an epidural. However, things were not going so well and I needed to help. I was sliced from stem to stern and my poor baby was hauled into the world with the largest pair of salad servers I had ever seen. Her poor little face was a mass of bruises because she had been rammed face first into my pelvic bones for hours by the relentless contractions. My doctor apologised at my follow up appointment and said he absolutely should have performed a C-section and he should never have put the two of us through that ordeal. Then he finished with this elegant summation, "You may be bovine on the outside, but inside you're built like a chicken. The big-boned girls are like that sometimes, surprisingly inadequate."

I think I went into a kind of dissociative state. I went through the motions, I smiled at the visitors and laughed as all the aunts and grandparents argued about what the best way to take care of a baby was. I was connected to none of it as I floated just outside of my body observing it all. Once again, I donned a mask, *perfect mother*, and behind it I lived in abject terror. What the hell did a perfect mother even act like? I wouldn't know one if she came up and bit me in the arse. I hadn't thought as far as having an actual baby! Mythical baby, yes. I'm pregnant, yes. When's baby due, yes. Actual real live breathing, bruised, jaundiced baby that would be wholly dependent on me for… well everything, no. The enormity of the responsibility took my breath away. I had no resources to pull from. No example to follow. I was once again completely alone with a world of expectation crushing down on me and I'd missed the brief.

Thank God for strong maternal instincts that welled up seemingly from nowhere. The moment I held that battered little soul and looked into her eyes and saw her confusion and her fear, I knew that my mission in life would be to protect her from anything remotely resembling my childhood. She would know, without a shadow of doubt that she was loved and wanted and cherished. I wanted to hold her in my arms forever and never put her down. I think that moment of meeting my baby, was the first time in my entire life that I experienced real love. I swore to her that I would give everything I had to protect her and give her everything that life had denied me. That was the day my inner warrior woke up.

Apart from suffering through post-natal depression that caused me to give my baby away to my GP (a thoroughly nice man who could do a much better job that I could, he was surprised to hear when I trundled into his consulting room while he was busy with another patient and handed over my most precious baby), I handled motherhood like a pro.

A short stint in lockup, courtesy of the now not so nice GP, a few false starts and it all came together. Once someone took the time and trouble to explain what PND was about and I understood it properly, I stopped feeling like a possessed mad woman and put a plan in place so sort it out. I went to the gym and did three aerobics classes a day until my hormones straightened themselves out again. Simple!

Breastfeeding was another shocker. The morning I woke up to a full milk supply I thought I had been invaded by body snatchers. The size of the things on my chest! They started right under my chin and threatened to overwhelm me. Milk sprayed everywhere all day long and I'm still surprised to this day that my poor child didn't drown at the breast or develop a life-long fear of food. Two rounds of mastitis didn't help, but I pushed through and fed successfully for nine months. That's how parenting went for me, life set up a problem and I knocked it down and waited for the next one to appear. Nothing, but nothing, would hurt my child and she would have her every whim and desire taken care of, or I would die trying.

Three years later, my second child popped out onto the operating table after a twelve-hour trial of labour. She had the good grace to go into foetal distress necessitating a C-section thereby saving us both the horrors of natural childbirth by a *surprisingly inadequate* mother. I will always be grateful to her for that. I had the same experience with this little one, that feeling of complete and utter love and a fierce desire to protect and shield her. I still marvel today how these little souls arrive equipped with all the love that is needed to fit themselves right into your heart. I know that immediate bonding isn't the experience of every new mum and I apologise if that offends anyone, but huge wins have been few and far between in my life story and I am holding onto this one like a prize fighter holds their championship belt. I AM a loving mother, I've got this.

Did I do everything right? No. Did I make mistakes along the way? Hell yes. Did I do everything within my power to raise my girls right? Yes. Do I have regrets? Yes. Did I scar them in ways I couldn't begin to understand? Yes. Could I have done a better job? With the benefit of hindsight, yes. Was I a good mother? Yes. My girls always knew that they were loved, wanted and cherished. They have lived their lives with a warrior on their side. Our dance style was more thirty second dance party in celebration of being, achieving, trying, succeeding and taking part. I didn't care, I celebrated my girls from the bottom of my soul. They remain the thing I am most proud of in this life, my greatest achievement.

Life Lessons:

- Life can be lived on default settings
- Guardian angels are real
- I am surprisingly inadequate
- Love really does exist
- Knowledge is power
- I'm a good mother

Chapter 7

The health conundrum

Then the health issues started. I'd always suffered from sore throats, even after the removal of the tonsils and I had frequent bouts of bronchitis and pleurisy. Now however, I had a bone crushing tiredness and my joints ached. I had a weepy, painful rash across my face. I tried treatment after treatment, doctor after doctor, specialist after specialist, all to no avail. I even had a sleep study done after I started falling asleep at traffic lights whilst driving. Nothing. Nothing to do, but keep on keeping on, but always in the back of my mind was that niggle of doubt. Was there something wrong with me? Was I imagining it? How is it possible to imagine a wet, weepy rash on your face… everyone can see it! The very nice GP couldn't seem to get past the fact that I had once tried to give him my child and he cried depression every time I saw him. So, I stopped seeing him. I have found throughout my lifetime struggling with mystery symptoms, that when the medical profession sees a woman in trouble without obvious cause, such a bone sticking out of her leg, or blood gushing down her face, they automatically default to depression. Arseholes! (Remember that small, angry baby… she's still in there).

By the time my children were seven and four years old, it became clear that Husband and I could no longer continue together. We lived in total silence broken only by the chatter of the children. Communication between the two of us was non-existent. One fine day, after a ten-day period during which not one shared word was uttered (yes, I was counting), I stood in the supermarket trying to buy a lettuce. I was shaking and sweating and the panic was rising in me. The choice of which lettuce to buy was simply more than I could manage. Just as I felt that I was about to pass out, I heard a voice say to me, "So what do you want?" There was no one standing anywhere near me. I looked all round; my panic suspended. Nothing. Then I heard it again, as clear as day, "So what do you want?" I heard myself reply, "I want a divorce." So that's what happened. I drew up a long list of things I needed to run my own home, showed it to Husband and said if he couldn't see his way clear to facilitate that, I would stay, we would have a third child and I would never mention being unhappy again. He signed the cheque.

If talking heads of lettuce haven't clued you in already, here's where the weird shit portion of my journey begins. On one hand I was living my life, thirty years old and free for the first time ever. No Mother, no *them*, no Husband. I could explore anything, try out anything. I had no one to answer to and no one to censure me. On the other hand, I was living under a mantle of shame for having broken vows, I felt judged by everyone I knew, and I was consumed with guilt for hurting Husband and for rocking my children's worlds off their axis'. All change comes with consequences. I was having a coffee at a friend's house one day and she introduced me to her over-the-road neighbour. She was a little left of centre and certainly had qualities I didn't recognise, but there was something magnetic about her. She seemed to radiate... something! I was drawn to her in a strange way so when she invited me to join her meditation group, I didn't hesitate – well I did, I hesitated a lot but it sounds better in the retelling not to admit that.

Please understand I had no idea what meditation was having never been exposed to it in any way, shape or form. Off I trundled like a lamb to the slaughter. Turns out it was a group of people who sat or lay on the floor with their eyes closed, woo-woo music playing in the background, listening to the group leader drone on and on about Chakras and colours and caves and bubbles of love and goodness only knows what. Knowing that I had a knack for missing the brief, I sat quietly observing, waiting to see what would happen. After about twenty minutes, one by one, each member opened their eyes, stretched their limbs and *came back into the room* in line with the group leader's instruction. This was no problem for me of course, because I had gone exactly, nowhere. They sat up and they began to tell stories about what they had seen and done during the meditation. Oh, the stories they told. Riding on the backs of eagles they had soared across verdant plains; others had submerged their bodies in bubbling pools of coloured water; yet others had met with beings of such intense love that they wept, moved by the recounting of their experience. My mind was screaming, "Run! This is weird shit!! "I stayed put and no one seemed disappointed that I hadn't *had* an *experience*. They congratulated me on just allowing the relaxation energy to flow through me (Ok?) and they all seemed so happy. Something inside me was intrigued. I went back the next week.

My health was all over the place. I have had to put together comprehensive medical records to try and convince doctors I am not just an imaginative, depressive idiot. For the sake of brevity and to stop your eyes from rolling back in your head at my litany of woe, here's the cliff notes version. It's a real smorgasbord of misery, question marks and blind alleys (feel free to skip ahead):

- Childhood: Measles, sub clinical chicken pox, recurrent coughs, colds and tonsillitis. Tonsils removed aged 10
- Adolescence: From age 16 recurrent chest infections, bronchitis, pleurisy, boils – treated with various antibiotic therapies. Monthly migraines from first onset of menses
- Adult: Aged 21 had an ulcerative rash across nose and face treated unsuccessfully with antibiotics, Roaccutane, topical creams and UV therapy.
- Normal first pregnancy age 22 with forceps delivery. Probably the most well I have felt as an adult but suffered extreme fatigue post-partum – sleep study inconclusive. Post-partum depression treated with exercise and therapy.
- Viral encephalitis during pregnancy
- Less healthy second pregnancy, weight gain, migraines almost weekly, torn muscles around uterus – C-section delivery.
- Persistent, itchy rashes on tops of thighs, creases of arms and vulva. Biopsy inconclusive – treated unsuccessfully with various topical creams and UV therapy.
- Hacking unproductive cough 6 months+ diagnosed as irritable airways.
- Sciatic nerve pain.
- Ongoing migraines – allergic reaction to sulphur-based drug – facial numbness, tight chest, tingling in extremities, difficulty breathing. Treat migraines with Voltaren.
- Late 30's through early 40's – joint pain, ulcerative facial rash, fatigue – diagnosed with lupus despite negative ANA test. Treated with Hydroxychloroquine and cortisone for 8-10 years, during which time I was also given Methotrexate. That was subsequently stopped after scalp and facial shingles occurred.
- Slipped disc in back treated by chiropractor.
- Septicaemia from boil bursting inward requiring hospitalisation and antibiotic therapy.
- Developed tinnitus.
- Dislocated coccyx (dancing injury) – treated unsuccessfully with cortisone injection into tailbone. Pain for over ten years.

- Alternative practitioners challenged diagnosis of lupus in favour of adrenal fatigue and hypoactive thyroid – treated with supplements as thyroid tests remained normal.
- Surgical treatment of tortioned ovarian cyst.
- Diagnosed with polymyalgia arthritica – treated with cortisone.
- Weight gain out of control – unable to lose weight, alternative practitioners again suggested under active thyroid – treated with supplements as medical tests still normal.
- Menses stopped altogether around mid-40's. No symptoms of menopause experienced.
- Onset of seasonal asthma at around age 40, requiring annual hospitalisation three years running and treatment with steroids and bronchial dilators.
- Chronic persistent cough treated with Physeptone – had allergic reaction to this with psychosis and visual disturbances.
- Burning pain in feet with petechial rash
- Challenged rheumatologist diagnosis and he said probably not lupus. Dropped the Hydroxychloroquine but found needed to stay on cortisone to function.
- Diagnosed with heavy metal toxicity by alternative practitioner and treated with supplements.
- Large vaginal mass resulted in surgery to remove Bartholin's gland which was attached to a large chocolate cyst.
- Recurring mouth abscesses requiring antibiotics. Had allergic reaction to Myprodol – facial numbness, vertigo, spacial distortion. GP decided opioid allergy at play.
- Developed sudden allergy to macadamia nuts, facial tingling, hot flushes, tight chest and inability to breathe. Treated with cortisone.
- 2012 Fell down 4.5m embankment – broke big toes in both feet, fractured L1 vertebra, concussion, tore muscles along sternum.
- 2013 Recurrent chest infections – diagnosed as COPD. Was cautioned to wean off cortisone tablets and use preventative inhalers instead.
- Chest pains – had stress ECG results inconclusive except for hypertension.

Weird Shit!

- Diagnosed with Fibromyalgia
- 2014 Adrenal fatigue diagnosed by endocrinologist – weaned off cortisone and treated with cortisol. No improvement.
- Sleep study showed 23 apnoea episodes occurring every hour. Could not tolerate CPAP mask which induced panic attacks.
- 2015 Struggling with extreme fatigue, chronic insomnia, constant flu-like symptoms, tremor and aphasia, took retrenchment package and spent almost 12 months in bed. Rehabilitated by walking and swimming and multi vitamin and multi mineral supplements. Functional at around 20% capacity, but unable to work due to fatigue, pain and inability to concentrate well and poor sleeping patterns leading to exhaustion. Difficulty exercising due to pain, shortness of breath and legs go numb after +- 10 minutes walking.
- 2016 Experienced sudden weight loss – 10 kg in a month – at which stage the sleep apnoea stopped.
- Dental work done to remove/rebuild 4 broken teeth and replace 12 amalgam fillings over 4 sessions. Had a bad shock-like reaction to fourth anaesthetic.
- Cataracts in both eyes removed surgically. Had a bad reaction to the first anaesthetic, panic attacks and elevated anxiety. Gained 13kg in two weeks – sleep apnoea returned. Second cataract operation went off well.
- Currently 50kg overweight and unable to shift it.
- Migraines stopped almost completely since ceasing work and now occur only once or twice a year.
- 2017 Tested negative for Rickettsia and Lyme diseases, but test showed past exposure to Epstein Barr virus, cytomegalovirus, mycoplasma pneumonia and chlamydia pneumonia.
- Bone density scan showed osteopenia in spine
- Bad ear infection led to cellulitis of face and scalp requiring antibiotic treatment.
- Suffered PTSD following big shock, anxiety attacks, palpitations, tremor, excessive sweating, chest pains and facial numbness. All tests clear, but slightly elevated cholesterol and very high blood pressure. MRI – neurosurgeon identified four white flares on scan and queried MS and raised intercranial pressure. Neurologist however decided nothing wrong.

- Multiple kidney stones surgically removed. Due to previous allergic reactions no opioids given. Reacted poorly to first anaesthetic for insertion of uretal stent, but second op to blast and remove stones went well.
- Underwent genetic testing by dietician and was told I need to eat a low-fat diet; have slight methylation problems; need 8 hours sleep per night; and lots of high energy exercise. Exercise a major problem so went on a vegan diet for three months, which triggered gut symptoms of pain, bloating, flatulence and weight gain. Eye muscles twitching and blurry vision increased and fatigue elevated.
- Went for a colonoscopy as abdomen distended and rigid. Bowels not working. Conscious sedation, no opioids, surgeon abandoned procedure a third of the way through as I was apparently not tolerating the pain. He removed three large polyps and identified diverticulosis. Bowel was tortioned and twisted on itself. Recommended to complete procedure under general anaesthetic.
- Began an ongoing sinus infection. Treated with multiple antibiotics. ENT eventually put me onto strongest antibiotic possible plus cortisone. I ended up in the A&E with racing heart, chest pains, excessive sweating. ECG normal, treated with Ativan to correct nervous system overstimulation from the cortisone.
- Sinuses continue to flare regularly. Have stopped antibiotics as don't help, taking daily antihistamines.
- 2018 Was sitting on the floor painting furniture. Pulled out a heavy drawer and twisted around to put it on the bed behind me and something went horribly wrong. Couldn't stand or sit, horrendous pain. Had physio come to the house and she diagnosed psoas muscle injury. Treatment ongoing for 18 months.
- Frequent sinus infection, shortness of breath, hip and lower back pain. Burning feet, muscle spasms, extreme fatigue.

Life Lessons:

- I'm a wreck
- I think I'm drawn to weird shit
- Doctors are of no use to me
- I am once again alone

Part 2

Exploring the world of weird shit!

Chapter 8

The meditation vs therapy conundrum

Mother was a royal pain in my backside. The parents had relocated to be near me (why????) and I had found them a lovely apartment nearby. There were gorgeous gardens to wander in, safe and secure, an extra room so the grandkids could visit. It was affordable, warm, sunny... it was lovely. I painted the walls and hired a floor sander. I re-varnished the parquet flooring for them so it would be lighter and brighter and good and clean and fresh. What I forgot however, was to have the neighbours shot. Mother hated the neighbours and she seemed to think that they were all in collusion with *them. They* were still around. No longer a child, I found *them* more annoying and aggravating than frightening and I did my level best to ignore *them* and, as far as possible, her. However, ignoring Mother was like trying to keep your head above quicksand. She would grab you in and pull you under and the more you fought her, the faster you went down.

She was morally outraged that I had had the temerity to leave Husband and she made it her business to remind me as often as possible how lucky I was that anyone, let alone a doctor, had even wanted to marry me in the first place. I should be ashamed of myself for ever thinking I could do better and I was nothing but a trumped-up tart. She had known I was nothing but trouble from the get-go. She told me again and again how awful I had been as a child and how lucky I was that anyone had wanted me, but since I had made my bed, I would damned well have to lie in it! When you hear all of that venom every time you see your Mother and especially when it is delivered in a whisper out of earshot of the rest of the family, or with a big smile on her face so everyone else thinks you're having a nice chat, or horror of horrors, in a baby sing song voice while she is bouncing your pride and joy on her evil lap, it gets old very quickly. I made it my business to smile and pretend we were discussing the weather, or my children's cuteness. I guess I was complicit since I allowed her to continue, but it had been ingrained in me not to fight back.

Incredibly, she was wonderful with my children. She held them and sang to them; she read to them and ran around the garden playing soccer with them. She laughed at their silliness and clapped at their achievements. She told anyone she could how proud she was of them and how wonderful they were and how lucky I was to have such wonderful children. Perhaps she saw them as mini versions of their father and disassociated them from me entirely. Whatever it was, she was a loving nanna. It didn't last though and when they got to their teens, she showed them a snippet or two of her true colours. I can't think for one moment they liked it. They asked a friend of mine to come and rescue them once; I had gone away for a weekend and they were staying with her. Even my strong male friend was a little daunted at the prospect of having to tackle her. She was a formidable old bitch disguised as a warm, smiling grandmother, until you crossed her. I knew beyond a shadow of doubt that there wasn't a person alive who would believe me if I told them how she treated me. That theme has played itself out throughout my life in many significant relationships. I have got to learn to say No!

In light of my ongoing inability to stand up for myself against the united onslaught of Mother and *them*, I decided to try a spot of therapy. For someone who had hidden in plain sight their whole life, deciding to subject myself to scrutiny by a professional dealing in matters of the mind was not an easy thing, but I was desperate. It was imperative that I sort things out because I needed to protect my children and in order to do that, I had to keep my feet under me and be able to stand strong. The therapist, looking back, was perhaps the most ordinary of ordinary people I have ever had the displeasure of encountering. She was a bad fit for me and it seemed as though she was colluding with *them*. She spent every session telling me how I might improve my attitude and behaviour so that I didn't vex Mother. This was about the same time I started with the meditation group.

I had kept going back to the group and had become quite good at breathing in rhythm with the leader's instructions. One evening as I lay on the floor with my eyes closed, slowly breathing in happy air… and breathing out crappy air, I suddenly felt everything swirling around me. Behind my eyelids exploded a black, purple and green kaleidoscope almost like the aroura borealis (Northern Lights). I was intrigued. I turned my focus to this incredible light show, and as simply as that, my imagination caught fire. Circa *Alice in Wonderland,* I found myself walking along a path in a green field and I was going exactly where the group leader was guiding us to go. It didn't feel like I was watching a movie, it truly felt as though I was physically there. I walked along a path towards a tree and there in the shade, stood an enormous eagle. I climbed onto his back and I marvelled at how soft his feathers felt against my legs as he took off. He flew over that green field and it was so verdant it defied description. Suddenly the scene changed and we were flying over a sea of yellow flowers, like a canola field in the spring. I didn't have a second to think about how weird this all was. I was totally caught up in the moment and the pure unadulterated joy I felt was like being caressed. The scene changed again and we flew over an orange grove. The trees were pregnant with luscious oranges and my mouth watered as I marvelled at their plumpness, but I could not touch the fruit. Yet again the scene changed and we were flying over a barren landscape. This wasn't a nice place at all and I didn't like the feel of it. It felt unsafe and threatening. The group leader was talking about flowing red rivers and pink fluffy clouds, but as hard as I tried, I couldn't see anything red in this god-forsaken, awful place. I desperately wanted to be anywhere but there. I forced my eyes open and jumped up, just as the curtain blew away from the open window of the room and a large gecko dropped onto my shoulder. I confess I created a bit, I shrieked and completely harshed everyone else's buzz. I was completely at sea. What the fuck had just happened to me? Were there drugs in the tea cakes? What had I just experienced? But most importantly… how could I do it again?

I couldn't wait for my next therapy session to discuss this incredible turn of events. I wanted her to explain to me how meditation worked; what the process was in the brain that allowed one to be transported to a different place and time; to experience things in such glorious technicolour, so vividly and with such feeling. My mind was a tilter-whirl of questions. I was dizzy with excitement and I needed to know more. Well, I did say that no one would believe me if I spoke out about Mother's vicious verbal attacks behind her smiling face, didn't I? Well my excited recounting of the meditation experience went down pretty much along those same lines. This ignorant idiot looked at me in abject horror as though I was completely insane. She physically recoiled from me and the look on her face said it all. She was mute with disbelief. I left.

My inner ten-month old was by this stage in life quite adept at yelling "Well, fuck you too!" to anyone who I thought wasn't treating me right. It all happened quietly inside my head, you understand, but anyone whose actions seemed to confirm that they too thought I should be invisible, or that I was a failure, or I wasn't worthy, or who questioned my intelligence, who tried to limit me, anyone who was a bully, who ignored me… pretty much anyone in fact. I must say here, that words were not required for this confirmation. Me thinking they thought those things was grounds enough. I became in my mind, a one-woman commando unit whose sole purpose was to fight for the under-dog... me. I was a seething mass of righteous indignation and I was pissed off! Why the hell was I such an aberration to people. Why did I have to hide behind this mask of people pleasing, arse-kissing, agreeable, service-oriented doormat in order to be found acceptable? I had a power surging through me that longed to get out and I was too afraid to allow that to happen. I never felt quite safe enough to expose myself, but I had found meditation and in those precious moments I could be Helen of Troy, I could be Joan of Arc, I could be pretty much anyone or anything I wanted to be. I could feel sensual and desirable. I could feel powerful and in control. I could feel valued and respected. Somehow though, I could never manage to feel loved and wanted. That remained elusive even in the glorious magnificence that was my imagination. I simply had no frame of reference to draw from.

I was terribly excited. We were having a weekend long meditation retreat and others from outside of our group would be joining us. This was to be the first time I had encountered others like us. (Weird people who like to listen to woo-woo music and lie on the floor so they could float away in their heads and imagine weird shit!) There was a charged undercurrent in the gathering. People were talking quietly and a few times I heard the word channelling mentioned. Well I had no idea what that might be, but I was confident in my meditation skills and knew I could handle anything that came up. I felt quite shy around the strangers and hid quietly behind my invisibility shield whilst smiling and offering tea and sandwiches around. Come time for the first group meditation and we have some new elements at play. One of the strangers, a beautiful blond woman with a willowy figure, dressed in loose, flowing, hippy-ish clothing had brought along incense and a Tibetan singing bowl. She spoke in a soft, melodious whisper and seemed really quite lovely. I smiled in my mind as I imagined the bowl breaking out into a Frank Sinatra croon. Oh well, I would just have to wait and see what this was all about. The incense was lit and it was kind of hinky-smelling. Woody but sweet at the same time, a bit cloying. I wasn't sure I cared for it. I began to feel annoyed. Who were these people who had come into my sacred, safe space and were taking control, making me feel uncomfortable? My inner ten-month old stirred and my inner warrior quietly laid her hand on her sword.

We settled ourselves comfortably, as the blond woman stirred a wooden stick around the inside of the Tibetan bowl. Strangely, the sound it made was reminiscent of singing and was oddly soothing. We closed our eyes and our usual group leader (thank goodness) started to lead us into a meditative state. I'll be honest, I have no idea where we went or what we did, because all I remember was feeling a tap on my shoulder. I opened my eyes and the blond woman was kneeling next to me, swaying slightly. I started and our group leader came over and knelt on my other side. I was starting to sweat. Was this how it all ended? I was to be sacrificed in some weird ceremony I had inadvertently stumbled into. I started to struggle to sit up, but she put her hand on my shoulder and I instantly felt filled with a quiet calm. My heartbeat returned to normal and I almost began to feel good again... until she opened her pretty mouth and spoke in a Jamaican-sounding male voice and said, "We were wondering when you would show up. It's taken you long enough. Welcome."

Life Lessons:

- Meditation is a great way to take yourself out of your reality and give yourself a short break from the misery of your day to day life
- Therapy is a waste of time
- If you play with fire, you might just get burned!!!

Chapter 9

An orphan's conundrum

I gave meditation a very wide berth after that incident. I bowed out as graciously as I could (fled for my life) and didn't rush to go back. I had other things on my plate anyway. My Dad wasn't doing too well. A few years back they had admitted to me that they had run out of money. Their primary source of income was a British pension and the Rand just happened to be at an all-time strong point and they were in trouble. Whether it was the cortisone I was on to treat the lupus that made me brave or what it was, I'll never know, but I went out one Sunday and bought them a little garden apartment to live in. I saw it in the paper, toddled off just to have a look and an hour later it was mine; subject to bank loans of course. I was rather surprised at my moxie; I mean people like us don't own property. We rent other people's homes, fix them up, plant pretty gardens and then move again a year later when they get sold… every single year of our lives as a child, that was the routine. Now however, in their late seventies, my parents finally had a home from which they need never move again.

You'd think that might have softened Mother a bit and quietened *them* down but no, it seemed to incense *them* that I had made this grand gesture. She complained about the neighbours and muttered and grumbled and generally became an even greater trial than usual. Dad however, looked like the weight of the world had been taken off his shoulders and for that reason alone I shall never regret buying that little place. True to form, he planted a pretty garden, Mother continued to hate the neighbours and we all poddled along in our own way.

Dad started getting a lot of pain in his back. I took him to my chiropractor, the one who had kept me out of hospital when I slipped a disc mowing the lawn. Nothing seemed to help and so I took him to the hospital for some x-rays. He was ages in there, but I wasn't overly concerned, it was a busy hospital and I just figured he'd gotten caught in a queue. Some hours later a nurse came to call me and asked me to step into the cubicle with my Dad and the doctor. Dad had had a small melanoma removed from his eyelid a year or so prior. Apparently that tiny little brown dot had set off a catastrophic chain of cancers inside of my poor Dad's body and it had spread everywhere. Spine, lungs, liver and brain. Dad sat there stoically listening as we were told there was nothing to be done. There's nothing quite as impressive as a British stiff upper lip. I didn't know what to do, I didn't know how to breathe. I didn't want to look at my Dad because then I would have to accept that it was true. A long silence ensued, broken by Dad with these words, "Let's not tell your Mother. I don't want to upset her. I won't have any treatment. She won't manage. I'll just tough it out when the time comes."

He would rather die of untreated cancer than upset my Mother! I hated her more in that moment than I knew it was possible to hate anyone. My inner warrior picked up her sword and went to town. She sliced and diced and hacked her way through the myriad cords that bound us together, shrieking a primal warrior's roar! Just like that, I cut myself off from her. I separated myself from anything remotely resembling a connection and I disowned and disallowed her. She was nothing to me anymore. In that moment of shock, I took back my power from her and she ceased to rule my world... and she could bloody well take *them* with her! She would be physically taken care of, that's it. If she were a stray dog, I would feed her, so I vowed to do that for her and no more. I took probably the deepest breath I have ever taken and I turned to my Dad and agreed to be complicit in his silence. I hugged him and said I would do everything I could to help him keep this demon invisible for as long as possible and I would protect him from her as best I could.

We drove home in silence. We were halfway there when I heard Dad groan. I stopped the car and his face was convulsed with pain. He finally allowed himself to admit how he was feeling and as his last bit of resistance and strength crumbled inside him, he folded like a house of cards. He groaned and he rocked, he was in agony. I drove straight to ex-Husband's practice and ran in to call him. He wasn't there, but his partner came out and gave Dad a morphine injection in the car, he was in too much pain to get out. He whimpered as I drove him the rest of the way home. I wondered how I was going to get him out of the car and up the five steps to their apartment. The morphine had started to work a little by the time we arrived and as I opened his door our eyes met. Two warriors about to go into a battle neither of us knew how to fight. Cloaked in silence and muzzled for the sake of Mother's peace of mind, he nodded and took a breath and I helped him from the car. As he stood up his trousers fell down around his feet. I hadn't thought to pull up his zip and fasten his belt after the injection. One of the little old ladies that lived in the complex saw us and started muttering furiously, clearly offended at seeing my Dad standing in his underwear. At that moment I hated the neighbours too. What a pathetic sight. It broke my heart to see this brave and beautiful man subjected to such humiliation. I quickly sorted him out and we linked arms, took another big breath and climbed those five stairs together. The outward picture was of a father and his daughter arm in arm, strolling homeward for the evening.

He lasted exactly ten days. Every day he disappeared a little more as more faculties deserted him. He couldn't stand, he couldn't see, he couldn't clean himself. He had a horrendous hacking cough by now and the slightest movement caused him to whimper in pain. All Mother could focus on was that he not wet the bed or cough phlegm on her carpet. I ignored her as best I could. I had my two girls at home and I was working full time. I couldn't leave him in Mother's clutches so I hired a nurse to help him and to keep her at bay. In retrospect I believe it was cruel to keep her in the dark, but in that situation, he was all that mattered.

On the day after he lost his sight he started talking about his mother. He kept saying that she was there, standing at the end of his bed. I assumed it was the ramblings of a cancer ridden brain. On the tenth day I sat next to his bed stroking his hand listening to the deep and disgusting rattle emanating from the depths of his chest. I remembered how big and strong his hands used to seem when they were holding my little hand as we walked to the park where he would push me patiently for hours on the swings. I recalled how he saw me safely across the road and every time those gentle hands had picked me up when I had fallen. Suddenly, I was prompted to say the following words, "Enough Dad. It's time for you to go. You have nothing to fear. Where you are going there are gardens more beautiful than you could ever imagine. There are parks with bandstands and music so fine it makes you want to dance. There is freedom and light and everything will be wonderful. There will be no more pain. You can go Dad. I'll make sure she's taken care of. I'll do that for you. You can go now."

We all went home for dinner a little while later and we had barely opened the front door when the call came. The night Dad died, the lid came off of Mother's Pandora's box and it never went back on again. He had been holding her together with the strength of his love and without him, she was finished. It took her just over a year to die too.

Life Lessons:

- Sometimes you just have to take the plunge
- With an open heart, even enormous things are manageable
- No one can hurt you if you don't allow them to
- Cancer is a bitch

Chapter 10

The what to do with Mother conundrum

Somehow, we all got through the funeral, the house guests, the rituals that are so necessary for dealing with grief. As we went through the motions, they pulled us along on their steady tide and the days passed. Far too soon everyone had gone home and life intervened with its constant never-ending demanding for attention. Mother lobbied hard to come and stay with us, but I had made a solemn vow to my children years before that I would never allow her to live with us. I had to be strong and honour that vow. So, she stayed at home and for a while she seemed to do remarkably well. I popped in every day after work to check that she was eating and had everything she needed.

I need to back up a little here. Shortly after I bought the apartment for them to live in, Dad had needed to have open heart surgery. He had suffered with angina for as long as I could remember and it was time for a valve replacement. It was a risky venture given that he was eighty years old. I had taken Mother to visit him the day of the operation and when we arrived at the ICU there was a huge drama playing out. A doctor was astride a bed and was doing chest compressions, monitor alarms were ringing hysterically and everywhere people were rushing about and shouting. We waited outside until all had settled down again. The doctor came out of the ICU muttering, "That was a close call." Turns out it was Dad who was the object of everyone's attention. He had almost slipped the net and left us.

He suffered a morphine psychosis complication that caused him to speak in a very inappropriate manner to the nurses. It didn't last long and he was mortified when we teased him about it afterwards. Mother was horrified and decided she didn't want him back. He had embarrassed her beyond redemption. She wouldn't visit him again and would wait until he came home. Embarrassing Mother was a cardinal sin and I watched to see how that would play itself out and how long it would take. Once Dad had made a mammoth recovery and was walking up to five kilometres a day, she started acting out. She refused to eat. She wouldn't drink. She was insistent that the food would harm her and cause her pain in some way. She fell over all the time and had frequent episodes of mania caused by an electrolyte imbalance that landed her in hospital on more than one occasion.

One day I was at work when I had a disquieting feeling that something was wrong. It just wouldn't go away, so I skipped out to go and check on them. I found her lying on the floor face down and Dad sitting in his chair with his head in his hands weeping. He told me afterwards that when he looked up and saw me in the doorway, he thought he was looking into the face of an angel. She had fallen for the third time that day and he simply didn't have the strength to pick her up again. I think he was regretting not having slipped that net in the ICU. I hauled her up and we shipped her off to hospital yet again. Drip in place, she recovered quite nicely, until a Muslim lady was put into the ward alongside her. She was a prominent lady in the Muslim community or so I was told by the nurses. She wore her full burka regalia even in bed. The Imam and many visitors came each night to pray for her and Mother was terrified of them all. They were beyond her understanding and anything unfamiliar had a habit of sending her over the edge. One evening she announced in her famous stage whisper (that on a clear day could be heard three doors down), "They were throwing petrol bombs in the car park today. It was the Muslims what did it!" Well you can imagine my horror as every head around the lady's bed whipped around to glare at us. I assumed prayer hands and did a swirling finger gesture next to my head to let them know that she was insane and needed their prayers. They graciously nodded and returned their attentions to their patient. I went off in search of Mother's doctor. Something needed to be done about her and I was rooting for a lobotomy. We got her home again and she seemed restored. But something was brewing.

After Dad died, as I said, she coped rather well. When her campaign to live with us failed she changed tactics. I would get phone calls from her in the middle of the night. She was in a state of panic because *they* were coming in through the roof. I'd race around to the apartment and nothing was happening. Then she settled again for days and was quite lucid and level-headed and started lobbying me to live with us. I put it down to her being a manipulative old cow. One day I was sitting at the office and again had that feeling of dread; something was terribly wrong. I trundled over and found the apartment front door wide open. Music was blaring loudly (she never listed to music) and she had locked herself in the passage behind a security gate. She was sitting on a garden chair, with wads of cotton wool stuffed in her ears, the portable phone under her chin… and an axe in her hand. She appeared to be asleep.

Long, complicated story later, it turns out Mother was suffering from a condition called Paraphrenia which she had most likely had since I was born. It's likely the trauma of my birth was the catalyst for symptom onset and in retrospect it was no wonder she fixated her hatred and venom on me. I had always said there was enough material there for an entire psychiatric convention and it turns out I was right. Wikipedia defines it thus:

"Paraphrenia is a mental disorder characterized by an organized system of paranoid delusions with or without hallucinations (the positive symptoms of schizophrenia) and without deterioration of intellect or personality (its negative symptom)."

They were the auditory hallucinations she was having, and the poor woman was actually living in a state of perpetual fear of being found out and terror of being publicly exposed. Found out about what, I never discovered, but it appeared I wasn't the only one hiding in plain sight.

Well that changed the picture completely. She was dosed up with anti-psychotic meds, immediately had every side effect under the sun and became a living nightmare. It was clear she could no longer live alone and something would need to be done. She, however, no longer trusted me because I had ratted her out to the doctor and it was my fault she was now being *targeted*. I hired a nurse to watch her while I tried to come up with a plan. Any port in a storm being the order of the day, I went back to the hairy hypnotherapist to see if he could help me wrap my head around this new situation. His advice was sage and I have repeated it often to people in similar situations, He said, "Very few people wake up one day and admit they can no longer cope and need to be placed into care. You have a responsibility to ensure that she is safe and taken care of, not to mention medicated. Do your duty and stop dragging your heels."

The nursing home may as well have been the seventh circle of hell. She was inconsolable. I recall the day I told her she would be moving there. She looked at me with such venom and hatred and hissed at me like a snake. Then in a tone of voice that even in memory still turns my blood to ice she said, "Are you happy now? You have finally taken everything from me."

I still saw her every evening although by that stage she didn't know if she was Arthur or Martha. She would call me and whine, "I never go to your house anymore." I'd go straight round, get her ready, toddle her down the corridor one shuffling step at a time and fold her into the car. Then I would haul her out of the car, toddle her to the front door and settle her on my couch. I would go to the kitchen to put the kettle on and she would cry out, "No, it's not safe, I want to go back." So, I would turn off the kettle and do the whole process in reverse. Half an hour after I got home again the phone would ring… "I never come to your house". Middle of the night, "*They're* coming in through the roof." Argh!!!! She died of a heart attack a year later. When I got the call, I remember laughing and laughing and laughing. I was so relieved that it was finally over. A close friend of mine offered her condolences thus, "I'm sorry for your loss. I hope you aren't going to make a big thing out of it because you were never really close to her anyway."

Life Lessons:

- You never know what someone else is going through so be compassionate
- You are stronger than you think
- If you hang on long enough, it will end
- Other people hide in plain sight, it's not just me
- Always do your duty, even if it pains you to do so
- Keep your feelings to yourself

Chapter 11

The Reiki conundrum

A colleague gave me a voucher for a Reiki treatment. I hadn't heard of Reiki and didn't know what it was about but, I made an appointment and trundled off. I lay on a massage bed, fully clothed, woo-woo music was played softly in the background and the dreaded incense was lit. Sighing, I deciding to suffer through it in silence and I closed my eyes determined to drift off. I was exhausted. Burying parent number two had been a trying experience. The packing up of the home, the disposal of their earthly possessions and the execution of their last will and testaments, all the while running my home, dealing with the demands of two teenagers, working full time and on and on, had knocked the stuffing out of me. I still suffered terribly with joint pain and fatigue and I coughed for months on end. I felt like someone had removed my batteries.

The therapist placed her hands gently along my body in different positions and I was stunned at the incredible heat that was generated by her hands. Everywhere those hands went, I felt soothed and restored, like a crumpled pillowcase after it has been ironed. I liked Reiki! She told me it was a gentle healing therapy designed to reconnect the body with its divine light. Hey, I had been told I had the light, or was the light or something of that order and I was to shine my light brightly. Perhaps this was where I should focus my attention. No one spoke in a Jamaican lilt; I didn't have to do anything, just lie there and be ironed. I signed up to learn how to administer Usui Reiki.

I'm a big fan of cliff notes so here goes.

"Dr Usui, born in 1865, studied in a Buddhist monastery. He was interested in medicine, psychology and theology and was seeking a way to heal himself and others using the laying on of hands. He wanted to develop something unattached to any specific religion and religious belief, that would be accessible to everyone. He was on a meditative retreat, and after 21 days of fasting, meditation and prayer, he saw ancient Sanskrit symbols that he later used to create Usui Reiki."

I apologise profusely to all the great Reiki masters of the Universe for my limited and I suppose, somewhat disrespectful manner of describing this beautiful therapy. It isn't for me to educate people on your discipline. That is best left in the hands of the experts. However, that was my take home and I was intrigued. A healing modality that didn't involve doctors who historically had failed me on a grand scale, was something I was interested in. Also, this was a use of meditation I hadn't encountered before and I realised that in reality I knew nothing about anything to do with the subject.

As far as Reiki went, I was taught the positioning of the hands, the sequence that should be followed; and my goodness did my hands tingle and burn while I was doing it. This was weird shit in the extreme. Apparently, my hands had been activated by waving them around drawing those ancient symbols in the air. I didn't know about that, but I did the second course anyway. I refrained from getting the third and final Reiki Master qualification because I felt I simply didn't have the right amount of respect for the process. Firstly, I wasn't sure what this energy they spoke of was all about; where did it come from; who supplied it; could they guarantee it was safe to use? I wasn't in touch with any Gods or Universal deities, plus I had trust issues. I was assured that the application of Reiki energy was akin to pouring water into a glass of ice cubes. The energy got to where it was needed, regardless of the entry point. That being the case, I couldn't wrap my head around the requirement for strict adherence to hand positions and rigid sequences. Reiki does, however, remain one of my favourite therapies and if I ever feel like I need a good straightening out, I go and get ironed.

Life Lessons:

- There's no escaping your duties
- Regardless of how you feel, get up, dress up and show up
- Just because you can do something, doesn't mean you should

Chapter 12

The psychic vs medium conundrum

I have visited many psychics over the years and each one has stunned me with what they have said. This is weird shit on a whole new level. The first one I went to on a dare. Mother had often told us about the day she had her fortune told. She had gone with two friends to visit a gypsy fortune teller in London. They were surprised when, as the first lady sat down, she paused and said to them, "I write it down and place in envelope. You read later." No chit chat or questions would be entertained. After all the readings were done, Mother grabbed the three envelopes and they dashed off to a tea shop across the road to read their fortune cards and compare notes. An out of control car came around the corner and mounted the pavement killing one of the ladies instantly. A long time later, Mother was tidying out her handbag and she came upon the three envelopes. Fortunes cast aside and forgotten in the face of the harsh reality of bereavement. She opened her late friend's card and it was blank. The gypsy had seen that she had no future.

As you can imagine that put the wind up me good and proper. I'm not keen on exposing myself to scary weird shit, but I was dared to go and see one particular guy so off I trundled. He was quite well known in certain circles and was apparently really good. In for a penny in for a pound, off I went. I waited in his apartment lounge surrounded by an extraordinary amount of clutter and at least seven cats that I could see. The place stank of cat's pee and I was not comfortable at all. But like an idiot I sat there anyway and waited my turn. Good instincts (get the hell out of here), no ears (listen to your instincts)! Anyway, when the client came out, he looked like a normal person, was wearing a good suit and seemed in no way creepy, plus he seemed delighted and was thanking yon psychic profusely and pumping his hand enthusiastically.

I stood, smiled and entered the inner sanctum which was a dark, dingey room swathed with scarves and exotic fabrics. A salt lamp burned in the corner providing the only light source. The window was covered in dark black velvet curtains that blocked out all light. Himalayan flags adorned every surface and the wretched incense was burning like billio in the corner. Before I could flee, without even looking at me, he jiggled a little velvet bag and shook out onto the table an assortment of small bones. What the fuck?! Now what had I got myself into? Mother also used to say curiosity killed the cat and at this point I was afraid she might be right.

This strange little man launched himself into an impressively accurate story about my life and my circumstances; and I can honestly tell you there is NO way he could have known all that about me, not even if I had been followed by a private investigator. He knew what I thought, he knew how I felt. He saw right through my invisibility shield and he laid me bare. He peered at my shocked face and he chuckled. "Serves you right for taking so long", he said. Next, he shuffled some extraordinarily beautiful, if somewhat tatty looking tarot cards. I divided the deck and moved the cards around as instructed. He went on exposing me for the fraud I was. I began to understand the song *Killing me Softly…* with his words. He knew about my health, my symptoms, my deepest secrets, everything I made it my business to hide from the world. It was so creepy, like looking into one of those distorted mirrors at the fun fair. My ears burned and my heart pounded. I longed to run, but I couldn't move. Then he began turning over some circular cards and told me I would be travelling over the sea within a three. I'm not sure what within a three meant, but I did know that at that stage in my life I didn't have enough money to travel up the road let alone over the sea, so I started to relax as I reassured myself he was a fraud. Then he picked up a small crystal ball. He peered in and started to chuckle. "If you don't clean that green swimming pool of yours, you won't be able to swim. Take care of your business, stop dragging your heels." My pool looked like a duck pond! Then he stood up and ushered me out and I know for a fact the expression on my face was gormless. I went home and cleaned the pool. Three days later a friend called me to ask if I wanted to go to London for a three-day weekend. She had won some tickets. We were to leave in three weeks.

As I say I have seen many psychics since then. They are not all weirdos who live in cave apartments, drowning in cats. Some of them are perfectly regular looking folk who are professional with a capital P. Each one of them has always given me something precious in their messages, something relevant that I needed to hear at the time. Without realising it, I was slowly allowing myself to accept that there was something else out there and I was allowing myself to have faith and trust them. The really good ones had a common language, they all told me their messages came from Spirit and that only the highest good would be served by their messages. So, whilst I didn't fully appreciate what that meant, I liked the notion of a highest good, and I allowed myself to be comforted by the words. I continue to see psychics from time to time for clarity on some conundrum or other that I am wrestling with.

My all-time favourite medium touched me so deeply that I ended up doing two workshops on psychic development with her. She has to be the clearest conduit and the most ethical lady I have met. Her messages come through clearly without a trace of ego. I went to see her a short while after Dad passed away. I was drowning in Mother's madness and I was looking for motivation to keep going. She hadn't met me before and she asked no questions and did nothing other than open with a most beautiful prayer to the blessed Mother, Father, God, for our protection; and a call for both of our Spirit Guides to step forward and guide the messages. I have Spirit Guides?! Really? Who knew? Her opening gambit was, "I have a gentleman stepping forward, he's so lovely and cuddly, I think he's your Dad. He wants you to know that you were right, the gardens are so beautiful and there are bandstands that play music." I was immediately reconnected with the promise I'd made to Dad on his deathbed, that I would look after Mother for him so that he could go. I found the reserves I needed to go on.

The psychic development workshops were next level weird, but by this stage I was just going with the flow. We sat in comfy armchairs in a lovely room, there was no woo-woo music and no incense. It was all so wonderfully normal. I was keen to learn as much as I could about this all-knowing, wise and comforting Mother, Father, God, Spirit, Other side, whatever it was called. I shall refer to this as Upstairs from now on. I learned that we are all energy and that energy can change form. We have energy centres in our bodies called chakras. Each chakra is assigned a colour and a purpose; I'll explain more about that in part three. Our purpose on the workshop was to learn to listen to our intuition. Then she surprised me by saying that everything we would learn, we already knew. She would simply help us to reconnect with our wisdom, like opening the shutters on the library shelves so the knowledge could flow out. She told us that in the world of metaphysics, which was the space we were now entering, all knowledge resides. She explained that we were spiritual beings having a human experience. We built ourselves a blueprint for our lifetime designed to help us learn a lesson, achieve a goal, master an aspect of humanity, or work out a karma. We had a primary karma that we came to Earth to deal with.

I have heard all of this information repeated by so many different authors, resources and teachers, but I shall credit them to this lady because she was the first to respectfully answer my many questions. Apparently, we are part of a large soul family. Souls travel in large groups. From within that group we select the cast to play out the blueprint we have designed for our lives. I was fascinated. The other thing that I was stunned to learn is that you can come back again and again and again until you master your lesson or achieve your objective. Then you can choose to come back and learn something else, or you can stay in Spirit and help others out remotely. Now I was a corporate girl by this stage in life and this resonated so powerfully with me my head almost exploded.

Look at this and see how neatly it all fits together.

- Define your purpose – master self-worth
- Build a strategic plan – decide which life you want to live
- Create a project plan – draw up life blueprint
- Engage resources – Either engage a cast of characters that will validate my self-worth (lesson achieved – the easy way); or engage villains who deny me any validation forcing me to seek out my own self-worth against all evidence to the contrary (the hard way).
- Assign project manager – hook up with spirit guide
- Put in safety measures – assign guardian angels
- Launch plan – be born

Life Lessons:

- At a certain stage in your journey going back is no longer an option
- Curiosity energises the cat
- Always find trustworthy, genuine, professional teachers without ego issues
- Everything in life is the same, just variations on a theme

Chapter 13

The tarot card conundrum

The wonderful medium suggested that I might consider a career in mediumship. She was confident that I was well suited to it and saw a lot of potential. However, the scars of my upbringing still held me back. Potential alone was insufficient to motivate me and I was not confident enough to put myself out there in such a manner. The world I lived in had no frame of reference for the weird shit I was learning and I knew that I would meet resistance, ridicule and disbelief from everyone I knew. I had children to raise and I was simply not brave enough to take the risk. I had insufficient connection to my self-worth to step outside of my comfort zone where I could be seen. So, the see saw continued. Up - you have potential; Down – who do you think you are, trumped up tart, filthy slut, surprisingly inadequate, no one will want you, people like us don't…

Seeing my struggle, she assured me I had the highest level of souls looking after me and I would be alright in the end as I was a much-loved soul. She recommended I see a lady who practised a discipline called Wholism Healing. I would be able to find her at a coffee shop run by a tarot reader. Tarot! My ears pricked up remembering the beautiful tatty cards that had magically sent me travelling overseas.

I tottered off to the Tarot shop and immediately forgot all about the Wholism Healing. I booked a tarot reading and once again, was blown away at the things the reader could tell me. I immediately signed up to do a tarot reading course. It was brilliant. I had my own deck of beautiful cards and I learned about what each one represented and what they all meant. I learned how they could be used to look at different aspects of a person's life and how the information was elicited from the person's energy field. Come time to read the tarot however and I discovered it held no appeal for me whatsoever. Once I knew how to do it, I no longer wanted to. Hmm!

Back to the drawing board. I was sitting having tea one day and the tarot teacher said, "Why don't you have a Wholism Healing session. Here comes the therapist now." Of course! That was what I had gone there to do in the first place.

Life Lessons:

- Nothing great ever happens in your comfort zone
- Stay focussed
- I'm a spiritual being having a human experience (?)

Chapter 14

The Wholism Healing conundrum

I don't remember my first appointment with this therapist, but it must have been a doozie because I signed up for two back to back sixteen-week courses that blew my mind completely. Have you ever thought about the fact that once you know something you can never un-know it and you are compelled to be someone entirely different? Well this one was a game changer. I learned to scan bodies with my hands. Not just bodies, but invisible bodies, we have more than one. I gathered information from chakras and cellular memories and I learned to trust my intuition. At last I found the courage of my convictions and when I heard or felt something, I spoke it. I learned to trust. The body on the bed always gasped and wanted to know how I knew what I was imparting. I was finally on the other side of the table. I will explain more about this weird shit in section three.

I began to consider a career as a therapist and I was keen to get in as much practice as I could. We learned about anatomy and physiology, energy, Spirit, chakras, and inner child. The inner child was the one that tripped me up every time so I skirted carefully around the issue of my own. However, I remember one profound session when we started to learn about it. I was working with a gentleman student who had a rugged, tough exterior. He was a manly man and he had it all going on. I was invited to read his inner child via his chakras and I jumped at the opportunity. The moment I put my hands into his energy field I was transported to a strange kitchen. The experience was very similar to meditation journeys. I had no idea where I was, but there was a little boy wearing a cowboy hat sitting on the floor playing with a puppy. I observed this happy little scene quietly. An adult male entered the kitchen. He was drunk and shouting abuse and the little boy grabbed his puppy and clutched it to him protectively. The wretched man was hurling abuse at the small child and was taunting him that, "Cowboys don't cry!" The little chap was sobbing in fear now. The man grabbed the puppy and wrung its neck! He threw the limp little body down on the floor next to the child and left shouting, "Cry about that you big baby!" I was horrified. The facilitator realised something big had gone down because she came over and called the session to a close and settled us all calmly again. There was no way I was recounting that tale to this chap. It was beyond hideous. She insisted I tell him, admonishing me that it was not my job to edit the information given by his Spirit Guides. It wasn't about me and if I had been shown something, then he needed to know. Taking the coward's way out I said in a tremulous voice, "Cowboys don't cry." That's all, nothing else. Well, what transpired next shocked me even more. This tough, rugged man came unglued in spectacular fashion. He wailed and wept, he cried and he sobbed. I sat there with huge eyes. What the fuck had I done? This shit was just too weird. The facilitator skilfully managed the situation and guided him back from his crisis and as he became calm again, he began to tell us the story. It was exactly as I had seen it. His father was an alcoholic. He taunted the boy for being soft. He had killed the puppy to punish the child for crying. That little boy had locked that memory up so tight, had plastered over it and had forgotten all about it. Fast forward to adulthood and you had a father in a locked horns battle with his six-year old son. The boy was desperate for a puppy and without knowing why, dad was ardently opposed to it. The son was beginning to withdraw from him and as a parent, he was stuck. Now however, he had the understanding he needed to make a different decision with his son.

This was a discipline I could work with. Answers came to me in story format. I could work with that. I could impart those to the client in as tactful and respectful way as possible and then help them understand the implications. The caveat to that, I always felt, should be that the client had to sign a waiver stating that should they become unduly distressed by anything revealed to them during a session, they agreed to seek counselling.

Every session there were more and more stories, all the same. Wounds uncovered, connections made, solutions presented and I learned not to attach to the outcome. I learned that the information was not mine, it was for the client. I did nothing other than connect the client with Upstairs being their Higher Self or Spirit Guide or the Universe or God or whoever was disseminating the information to them (we all believe different things). We always worked under protection of the highest good and we didn't dabble in anything dodgy. Weird, yes; dodgy, no! Imagine that the Universe at large is the energy source, the client is a lamp (seeking some form of light, be it to shine a light on a problem perhaps, or to lighten a burden they are carrying, or to lighten their spirits), the facilitator is nothing more than the plug that connects the two. She has no part to play beyond connection and possibly translation. Whether the lamp/client chooses to emit light, absorb light, allow light in is entirely up to them. Sometimes people can be so far removed from the reality of who they are, resulting from many wrong turns or mis steps along their life path, that it is difficult for them to light up. It's taken me many years. Surviving my life had somehow smashed all the lights in my existence and I had stumbled in the dark for most of it. Through this work though, I was beginning to see light again. Perhaps one day I would have the courage to let it shine brightly.

Life Lessons:

- No matter how far off course you are, you can always course correct
- So many people are hiding deep wounds, sometimes without even knowing it
- When you feel stuck in your life, there is always a reason
- It's best to be brave and face your fear
- We are all entitled to shine

Chapter 15

The rehab conundrum

Before you jump to the conclusion that I took up drinking or drugs… just no!!! One of my fellow students from the Wholism Healing courses managed to wangle the two of us in working at a drug and alcohol rehabilitation centre. She had gone along and pitched the idea of energy healing to them and initially they had drawn down the shutters on her. Undaunted she merrily said, "Fine, then let us work with your staff, I'm sure they could do with some healing." It worked and we were in. Every Saturday we'd arrive and the staff fought over the few allotted time slots. The staff gave such glowing reports to management about how beneficial they found the sessions that soon we were allowed to try it out with some of the clients. Understand that rehab is a very controlled environment and the clients are struggling. I have the utmost respect for anyone who manages to complete a stint in rehab. These troubled individuals with their varying addictions are taken apart and then carefully put back together again. Hopefully they came out with a better understanding of their condition and with new layers of coping skills. Sobriety is always a tenuous situation with the possibility of relapse ever present. The greatest irony for me is that the clients I worked with all felt as though they were broken remnants of the person they should have been; yet when I connected with their energy fields and their Higher Selves, they were some of the most magnificent, powerful individuals I have ever met. They had simply gone way off track. It was my utter privilege to have worked in that environment and I remain forever grateful for the opportunity.

We were sent the clients who were struggling with therapy. The resistant ones that weren't doing so well. I guess we became the any port in a storm port. A typical session in rehab went like this. The client would shuffle in, body language clearly letting me know how broken they were. Shoulders slumped, eyes downcast, voice slightly quavering, apologetic almost for their very existence. Either that or they burst in, belligerent, in full on defensive mode acting like they could take you down if they had to. I put them on a massage bed, explained what energy healing was in loose terms and opened with a prayer of protection. This was the point when they would tell me they were atheist, or there was no God. I would connect with their energy field and I would start seeing… cartoons in my mind, or I would hear nursery rhymes! Wtf? Now please understand that some of these guys were powerfully important businessmen with addiction problems. They were sometimes CEOs of massive organisations. Men used to wielding power… and I'm seeing fairy rings and dancing toadstools. Without breaking confidence in any way, I will share the stories of a few of my favourite clients. I do not know who these people were, what their names were, or where they fit into society. Often, they were in rehab under assumed names to protect their identity; plus, this was years ago. Their stories however, are common and demonstrate clearly the urgent need for self-knowledge.

The powerful man for whom I had picked up a fairy ring, was a challenge for me personally. Given that I am operating in the world of weird shit that ordinary folk are unfamiliar with, it can be tricky sometimes to interpret in a manner that isn't confrontational to them. I had been schooled and schooled hard, that it was not for me to edit information. I was to hand over what I picked up. So, I explained to this powerful man about the delicate fairy ring I had seen. He wailed and wept, he cried and generally broke down. It went back to his childhood when he had had a bad temper as a four-year old. His bossy elder sister gave him a tough time, probably suffering with sibling rivalry. He was the heir apparent and the fact that he was a boy gave him elevated status in the home. He knew from the time he could understand anything, that he would be a businessman like his dad and he would one day run the family empire. Well, his sister had built a fairy ring in the garden and in a fit of pique one day he had smashed it with a golf club. She promptly screamed at him that because of him all the fairies in the world had died and there could be no more joy. As a sensitive four-year old, albeit with a temper when aroused, he was devastated. He grew up feeling guilty and joyless. Since he had ruined joy for the whole world, then he couldn't allow himself to ever feel any joy. He hated business and wanted to be an artist, but his punishment for ruining joy was to become CEO and run the family empire. No wonder he was seeking spiritual comfort at the bottom of a bottle. I hope he took to heart my suggestion of painting on the weekends as a way of reconnecting with this true self.

I only ever saw a client once. Once was enough. Every time we managed to unearth the root cause of their addiction. That moment in their lives when they decided they were not worth saving. That moment that set them on the wrong path and changed their story. It was truly humbling. Often the most insignificant events were the catalyst for derailing an entire adult life. Most often they were completely unaware of what was at the root of their problem and that explains why they were struggling in therapy. They didn't know what to work with. The beauty of a rehab facility is that you can go straight to the cold face with a client knowing that they are in a 24/7 therapeutic environment where they will be held and helped as they come to terms with their truth.

I had a client one day who had *sad demeanour* emanating from his very core. He kind of oozed himself onto the bed, actual meaningful movement seemed beyond him. I was stunned when I connected with his energy field and felt him to be a vibrant, lively soul, upbeat and full of energy. Wondering how he had moved so far left of his centre, I asked his Higher Self for clarity. The only image I saw was of a couple standing at the alter on their wedding day. The bride had no face. Well that was a tricky one. I didn't know what had started his addiction to alcohol. Maybe he had been left at the altar. I needed to proceed cautiously. Then I broke all the rules and decided to ask him to tell me his story. I never did that because I didn't want to be influenced when I worked in the energy field. He told me he had attempted suicide a number of times. He had hooked up a hose pipe to the car and tried to gas himself, but his daughter was feeling sick and came home early from school. He then tried to hang himself, but the rope broke and he ended up with a broken ankle. He tried to shoot himself, but the gun jammed and he broke a tooth. He had tried to drive his car into a wall, but he forgot to leave his seatbelt off and so that didn't work either... the litany of woe went on and on all delivered in the saddest, smallest voice I had ever heard. And then I broke the rules again. I started to laugh. I laughed and laughed like a woman possessed. Nowhere in any counselling manual will you find the instruction to laugh at your client's pain, but I was rolling on the floor with tears pouring down my face. Eventually the sad narrative droned to a stop and he looked at me with a confused expression on his face. I heard myself say, "You are so stupid! You don't get it do you? You are not supposed to die!"

Shocked at my response, I made a concerted effort to pull myself together, but it was exactly what he needed. He suddenly broke out into a huge grin and said, "I'm the man that heaven didn't want." He liked that title. I did too because at least he was no longer identifying with his sad sack persona. He had pinked-up a bit if you will. He was so accustomed to people feeling sorry for him and when I had reacted so inappropriately it had short circuited his pattern of behaviour. I'm miserable, you feel sorry for me, misery squared. Crazy lady laughing at his pain... no pre-programmed response to that situation and so his brain had kicked into a different gear. As soon as he was out of his familiar woe-filled groove we could begin to work together.

I mentioned the wedding I had seen and the faceless bride. It turned out that the love of his life had been stricken with a mental illness that rendered her unrecognisable to anyone who knew her. She had receded into a world of her own and nothing and no one could reach her. She had been that way for over 30 years. They'd had exactly one year together as a married couple, just long enough for their daughter to be born, before this tragedy struck. He was drowning his sorrows with alcohol. He had the option of putting her into a care facility, but he couldn't allow himself to do so because he had made vows to her. I remembered the hairy therapist's advice and suggested that putting her into a safe and comfortable environment and paying for her care was in fact honouring his vows to her. He could free himself from this unbearable burden and let himself live again. His daughter was begging him to do just that, and his wife's doctors had said the she would never recover. He suddenly saw that his martyrdom wasn't helping her in any meaningful way and he was destroying himself in the process. The enormity of the decision to save himself was so great that he had chosen to die rather than face it. However, since heaven wasn't ready to admit him just yet... One always has to trust the information given. It is not for the facilitator to edit it.

"Ding dong bell, pussy's in the well". Well that's what I told the drug addicted young woman on the bed one day. She looked at me with the disdain of the youthful and let me know in no uncertain terms that I was a total whack job. Hey, only one of us was doing drugs, but potato, potahtoe. Carefully crafted conversation later, I discovered this young woman was from Namibia and had grown up in the heat of the desert. She was the pride of her school and had been sent to university in Cape Town. She would study some environmental courses that would allow her to make significant changes back at home that would benefit whole communities. She, however, couldn't adapt to the cold wet climate and was as miserable as a wet cat. Ding Dong Bell – school bell; Pussy's in the Well – not the right environment for a cat; Who put her in – her community had sent her to gather vital knowledge that she could take home to her right environment. In so doing she could become the hero she was born to be. She needed to stop soothing herself with drugs and find other means of dealing with her discomfort. She had a job to do and self-sabotage was not on the agenda. She got it. I hope she's as happy as a clam back at home, thriving and enriching the lives of entire desert communities.

The last story I'm going to share touched me deeply and taught me such an important lesson. This young man came into the treatment room flaunting some serious attitude. He wasn't going to take shit from no one and he was radiating warning signals. I thought, oh brilliant another tough guy. I had seen two combative characters already that day and was feeling a bit weary. He sat on the massage bed with his legs swinging and refused to lie down. Fine, I can work sitting up, the bed is non-essential to the process anyway. I asked him if I could put my hand on his arm and he reluctantly agreed, glaring at me all the while from behind his beautiful brown eyes. The moment I connected with his energy, I felt compelled to tuck him under my wing, to protect him, or to clutch him to me and never let him go. His energy was magnificent. He felt like every mother's dream child. This kid had the most enormous heart and his potential was almost without limit. I didn't pick up any of the usual nursery rhymes or childhood ditties. I was getting no clues at all from Upstairs.

I had no choice but to try and engage him in a conversation. Perhaps what I needed to know would emerge naturally. "Why are you in rehab?" I asked him. Well long violent outburst later, it turned out this young charmer had been *forced* into rehab by his parents. He was sixteen and his mother was terrified of losing him to his addiction. He was livid that he had been put in this situation against his will. It wasn't his fault that he was taking drugs and it wasn't a problem for him, so why was he being punished? Say what? "Who made you take drugs then?" I enquired, "Whose fault is it?" He seemed stunned by the prospect of owning his choices and he just glared at me sullenly. Turns out he had fallen into a rough crowd. They were the drug dealer component of his neighbourhood. I gather the plan was to get him hooked and then turn him into a dealer. These low-life types know just how to prey on vulnerable at-risk kids. What was his vulnerability I wondered? What had made them decide to woo him? Still getting no assistance from Upstairs, I asked him why he thought these guys were so cool. He said, and I'll never forget this, "Because they let me be me. I'm good enough for them just as I am."

I asked about his relationship with his father next. Clearly there was a complete disconnect here. He didn't see eye to eye with his dad at all. He was the opposite of what his father expected of him in every way. Dad was a manly man who liked to barbeque, drink beer and watch the game with his mates. The youngster was sensitive and was more inclined to meditation and music. He adored his mother, but he hated his father. His father told him repeatedly that he was a loser, that he would fail at everything in life, he would never amount to anything. He had hooked into this rough crowd as an act of rebellion and now he was indeed, well and truly hooked. The problem with this youngster was that he saw no problem with his drug use. He thought it made him tough and powerful, someone his dad could relate to. In reality he was operating pretty far left of his natural demeanour and he had become unrecognisable to his distraught mother. He was in fact playing out the exact role his father had cast him in, dismal failure and loser. I could tell he was not ready to get clean.

I felt compelled to try and impress upon him that he, and only he, was responsible for the choices he made. No one had forced him to take drugs. It was his decision and his choice and he needed to own that if he was ever to find his way back. I found myself saying to him, "Well as far as losers go, you are doing a great job, so actually you are pretty successful. Seems your dad is completely wrong about you. You're a huge success. Do you want to keep being a drug addict?" He did. "Well then that's fabulous. This is your decision and you are responsible for it, you and no one else. If you are sure that you want to be a drug addict then get out of here and do drugs until you are bursting with the experience. Take it as far as you can. Roll around in it and enjoy every moment. However, the day you decide it no longer fulfils you, it isn't a sustainable way of life and you want to make a different choice and become successful in another area, come back and we can help you with that." You cannot force sobriety on someone until they are ready to do what is required to attain it.

He completed his rehab program and went on with his drugging. The next time I saw him, was almost six months later. I recognised him instantly by his beautiful brown eyes, but everything else about him had changed. He was a shell of his previous self. He had been cautioned that in order to stay clean he had to stay away from the guys he did drugs with. Of course, he did no such thing and within days of his release he was back drugging as though he'd never left. Everything went belly up one night when he was raped and almost killed by his dealer. That was his rock bottom. He had to go that far before he could begin to come back to himself. He was now ready to make those changes. He was looking for a new way of being successful. Successful loser was no longer a sustainable option. This time Upstairs had plenty to tell him. I sometimes think of this gorgeous young man with the limitless potential and the beautiful brown eyes and I wonder if he ever found his way back.

I had the privilege of working with many wonderful people in rehab. I know that each of them was better off after our session than they were before. They left with an added layer of self-knowledge and a reconnection with their wholeness, their innate and absolute right to experience a joy-filled life. It all came crashing down one day though. I was chatting with a friend whose opinion I valued highly. I had decided to start showing this side of my life to a few trusted friends and see whether it was really safe for me to come out of hiding. I was telling her how thrilling I found this work and I gave her a couple of examples of the type of sessions I was dealing with. I looked to her eagerly for approval. She told me, "You are not qualified to be working with patients who need counselling. You are not a psychologist. You have absolutely no right to be doing this." I left the rehab the next day. In retrospect, if ever there was a time for a jolly good, "Well, fuck you too!" that was it. But my house was built on sand. I still didn't honestly believe in my right to be powerful, so I went back into hiding. It's not on her, please don't think I am saying that at all. She simply held up a mirror and as usual the picture was distorted. It's all on me.

Life Lesson:

- Trust yourself
- Listen to your intuition
- You can lead a horse to water, but you simply cannot make him drink
- Don't let someone else's opinion be more important than your own truth
- People like us don't do things like that
- You are strangely inadequate

Chapter 16

The expressive vs amiable conundrum

I threw myself into my corporate job. A friend had hired me to help her with some menial tasks on a project she was running. Unskilled stuff, like buying photographic props and filing. I worked a whole year without salary. I was only too happy to be included in this exciting world. At the end of the project, the CEO called me in and asked me why I hadn't wanted to be paid. I felt a bit foolish saying I was just happy to help. Remember, I'm the *service to school*-girl. He asked me if there was anything I really wanted and I was surprised to hear myself say, "A leather lounge suite." He told me to go and choose one and send him the bill. Well people like us didn't have leather lounge suites and frankly, I was stunned. Not only had the big boss seen me and thanked me for my contribution, he actually wanted to reward me for my efforts. Loyalty to this guy became the order of the day. I would do whatever this company wanted me to do, for as long as they wanted me to do it. That lasted over twenty years and yes, I did get paid.

But it wasn't my dream, or my passion, I was a player in someone else's dream. I became, externally, a stronger, tougher version of myself. I wore the mask as best I could and played the part expected. I worked twelve hours a day, six days a week. I stuck my nose in everywhere. I did every course they offered and wrapped my head around the rhythm of the corporate world. I discovered I loved process diagrams and flow charts, strategic mapping and tactical plans, reporting and analysis. I loved working out the best way to do things, plotting that as a process flow diagram, teaching others how to do it and managing the outputs. For someone who spent her whole life missing the brief and being confused, this was heaven. You were told exactly what was expected of you. You were given the tools to do the job and you were even measured and given positive feedback to help you do your job better. Plus, I was in a great environment where recognition was the culture and staff were rewarded for their contributions. Potential was spotted, picked up, nurtured and grown organically. I made work the most important thing in my life because for the first time, I was seen and given positive feedback. I developed a pretty unhealthy relationship with my job.

Yet I always felt like an imposter, a mask wearing wannabe. I had no qualifications. I hadn't gone to college or university. People like us didn't do things like that. I was once again running on pure instinct and my wits and in some cases sheer bloody mindedness and hard slog. Whilst it was thrilling, it was exhausting. I almost got found out as a great pretender when we did a personality styles workshop. Skinny cliff notes version: There are four main personality styles. Driver – Just do it! Expressive – Excited, let's make a noise about this; Analytical – Let me think it though; and Amiable – how can I help you get that done? You answer a questionnaire designed to discover whether you are more Task or People oriented; and more Ask or Tell. You end up with a double label, your secondary trait first and your primary trait second. Backup behaviour (that which you exhibit under duress or when you are right out of your comfort zone) is generally polar opposite to your essential style. We were learning this so we could improve communication. We could learn to deal with colleagues in a manner that would give us the best chance of getting what we wanted from one another. The result of this was that productivity would rise and we would all be happier and more efficient. I found this very useful. One of my colleagues was an Amiable-Analytical which meant his preferred method of receiving a job brief was to be given lots and lots of information, in a calm manner with emphasis on how his input would benefit the greater good and the importance of his participation. He then needed to be given lots of time to think it through, ruminate on it and once satisfied that he had understood it properly, he would produce amazing work. Well I tested as an Expressive-Expressive and our style is… not that. He and I became excellent work mates once we understood one another properly.

The course leader was also an Expressive. Since doing the Wholism Healing training, I found that I was always picking up undercurrents or moods. Things being said that weren't necessarily meant; or worse still, things meant that were not being said. I was very susceptible to the energy in a room, to the subtle nuances in conversations and tonal values. It was a bit exhausting sorting out the explicit from the implicit communications. But I digress. The Expressive facilitator, to my mind, made it perfectly clear that she valued the trait of the Expressive set most highly and found the Amiable lot quite sad and second rate. This caused me great distress because I felt she was being a bully (she also reminded me of Mother) and I really identified with the Amiable characteristics. I thought they were phenomenal people. They tend to work best under guidance and leadership. They don't like to be left out on their own in the cold. In a group dynamic they follow and support and are bloody hard working, salt of the earth, can't do without them people. So, I very Expressively defended my opinion that I should be classified as an Amiable, which earned me a lot of ragging and teasing that has lasted a couple of decades.

My Dad always said to me, "Your mouth will get you into trouble one day my girl." He was not wrong. Since retiring, I am happy to say that I stand by my statement and as I remove all my masks and learn to relax and allow myself to be who I truly feel I am, I will own an identity of Expressive-Amiable. A bit of an oxymoron I realise, but it fits me well.

Life Lessons:

- It's never too late to learn a new skill
- Perception is the mother of all devils
- I'm a loyal person
- I don't have my priorities straight

Chapter 17

The lupus conundrum

I had two priorities in life, my children and my job. I'm good at both. Looking back, if I'm completely honest, I did get the two muddled up and overemphasised the importance of work. In fact, I think my legacy to my girls was that I taught them how to be self-sacrificing workaholics. I shudder just saying that, but I have faith they will make much better choices in life than I did. Well I hope they will anyway. I had no time for personal growth or a personal life. I no longer meditated or prioritised joy; I just worked and worked and worked. My health was appalling although I could find no reason why. Many different specialists tried to fit me into the moulds of their particular learning. They ran tests with inconclusive results and when they couldn't provide a diagnosis, they were all happy to give me toxic medication to mask symptoms and send me on my merry way. No one seemed interested in finding out why I continued to be plagued with such a vast array of symptoms. I learned to hate the medical profession.

An interesting side note at this time is that I had a German Shepherd dog who had been diagnosed with lupus too. His belly skin was black and peeling and he smelt awful. He was a sickly dog and we weren't really close. My Border Collie, however, was an incredible little dog. He followed me everywhere and he gazed at me with adoration. The two of them were like two grumpy old men and they fought every single day of their lives. It was almost as if the sick and the healthy were battling it out for supremacy. I didn't make this connection until many years later. Both lived to a ripe old age; sadly, I had to put them to sleep on the same day. The GSD came into the lounge one afternoon and he slipped on the tiles. He couldn't get up by himself. I looked into his eyes and I knew what he was telling me. It was a Sunday so I promised to take him the next morning. I moved him onto his bed and we had a long night of chatting and making our peace with the impending situation. The next morning, when I let the Collie out, I noticed that he had bumped into the door jamb. He went out onto the driveway and sat staring up at the sky not moving. I rushed to him and his eyes were blue. I realised he could not see. I spoke to him and he didn't respond, he could not hear me. Tragically I had to load both of my boys into my car and go down and ruin the vet's day. He did say to me though that they wouldn't have been able to live without each other, they were so closely bonded. Even though they fought every day, they loved one another and were just simply my two grumpy old men. Losing both boys in one fell swoop gutted me and I was devastated. I grieved so hard for these boys and I wasn't sure I would ever get another dog.

After about ten years of being treated for lupus, I went in and challenged the diagnosis. I had umpteen alternative practitioners telling me I had adrenal or thyroid issues (even though the medical tests were always negative). I had this confirmed by Scio operators using fancy bio feedback Quantum something or other machines; pretty much anyone with a bio feedback mechanism on their laptop agreed; naturopaths, homeopaths, live blood analysts, iridologists, kinesiologists and every other "ologist" I could find. I had an astrologer run my natal chart and tell me there was no mark of the wolf in my constellations. Yes, I still dabble in weird shit, but only as a client. Lupus is marked by a butterfly rash across the face similar to the markings on a wolf which explains the astrologer's comment. The problem was, the supplements I was spending a fortune on with the *ologist* lot weren't helping me either.

My rheumatologist when challenged, said I most definitely did not have thyroid or adrenal issues because the test results were negative. I reminded him that the ANA test for lupus had been negative as well, but he had diagnosed it anyway. He turned around and said, "It probably isn't lupus, but I'm not worried about you. You can go can off treatment, you'll be fine." Now to juxtapose that statement, I am perpetually exhausted, some days even sitting up is challenging, every bone in my body aches, I have itchy rashes in places where the sun don't shine; I am plagued by boils and I cough and shake and sweat and wheeze continually. I cannot sleep properly, but I'll be fine. None of that concerns this esteemed specialist.

I'm not sure how anyone else would feel in a similar situation, but for me being labelled with a life limiting diagnosis was a pretty shit thing to happen. I struggled to come to terms with it. He had cautioned me not to do research or look it up on the web, but to simply listen to his advice. Every decision I made for those ten years was based on the fact that I was limited somehow. Not quite all there. A bit of a factory-reject if you will. Certainly, someone who should be grateful for anything she got, because frankly who would want to employ her, date her, love her, when she was less than whole. I made a conscious decision to never date again. I would not burden a man with this problem. I would stay focussed on my children and my work for as long as I was able to. The irony was not lost on me that an auto-immune disease where one's body attacks itself, had to be the purest expression of self-loathing. Maybe Mother was right, even my own body found me unacceptable.

I had decided to trust this man, especially when he gave me drugs that masked the symptoms, and I started to feel better initially. The reason for my challenging him all those years later was because the symptoms, whilst less vicious, had not disappeared and I still felt ill almost all of the time. Being told at that point that it was probably all a mistake, nearly blew my head off my shoulders. I did not know how to deal with this cavalier attitude. I felt betrayed at the highest level. I had trusted him!!! I was livid. I didn't see him again until about fifteen years later when by chance we were dining at the same restaurant. All credit goes to me that I did not get up and punch him in the face. I was still furious with him. It wasn't that he had taken a risk and treated something his instincts told him was at play contrary to test evidence; I almost respected him for that; I hated him for what I perceived as a lack of humility and humanity. These guys (and I am generalising here) do not seem to appreciate the power they have over their patients. They do not seem to understand that when they make a diagnosis, they could be changing the trajectory of their patients' lives. They seem to see patients as a collection of symptoms to be controlled rather than living souls with hopes and dreams and aspirations, who are seeking solutions and help. I have never found a medical practitioner who made me feel like I was anything other than… next! Body mechanics would be a more fitting collective.

So, there I was, completely at sea with no diagnosis to explain my troubles. I had a deep distrust of the medical profession and no clue where to turn next. What did I do? I sucked it up and toughed it out. Plastered a smile on my face, and I got on with life. I accepted less than as my lot in life, and I embraced my limitations. I also made an application to a local university to see whether I could enrol to study medicine. There had to be a better way, and even though people like us didn't do things like that, I was determined to find that better way. Unfortunately, because I had never been to a university, I could not join as a post grad plus, I was considered far too old for them to justify a slot in the programme. I would not have enough good years left to pay my debt to society for the privilege of having studied through their esteemed alumni. That was according to the woman I spoke to, who sounded a lot like Mother.

Life lessons:

- A sheep in wolf's clothing is just a sheep
- Sometimes you can lose everything in the blink of an eye
- It's too late, I missed the boat
- It is what it is

Chapter 18

The theatrical conundrum

So, there I was, still single, still gainfully employed, still ill, but faking it for all I was worth. I had concealed almost completely the extent of my suffering. Being around someone who is chronically ill seems to confront a lot of people. I was referred to as, oh mistress of ill health once by a colleague enquiring when I might get over myself and get back to work after I had needed a spot of sick leave. I'd had my sinuses washed out and this relatively simple procedure had knocked me right off my feet. I was weak and dizzy and disorientated and I was feeling utterly miserable. I could not seem to get my mojo back. After that sarcastic comment however, I began to feel insecure about my job, so I forced myself to get up and go back to work in spite of how awful I was feeling. I remembered that I should be grateful for what I had since none of it was earned, I was largely uneducated and I was really just lucky that anyone would want me at all. I simply pushed through.

Experience has taught me that people are either solutions driven, or they are totally fatalistic. The solutions guys will eat a burger, counter with a healthy walk, danger neutralised. Get cancer, have chemotherapy, survive or not, either way it is within the boundaries of what they know and understand. The fatalistic ones ignore all signs and symptoms, believing the great guy in the sky will sort it out for them and then they become surprised corpses when they drop dead. Have a chronic, unidentifiable disorder on the other hand... The fatalistic lot ignore you completely and just write you off as a whiner and the solutions people have no frame of reference for your peculiar situation. Some start treating you as a problem to be solved, the inference being that you are too stupid, too ignorant, or worse, too lazy to solve your own conundrum. Or they write you off as an attention seeking whack-a-doodle and apply what they deem to be the appropriate levels of disdain. I have spent a great deal of mental energy on this subject. This has helped me to understand the difference between empathy and sympathy.

Crude example: you break a leg. Anyone who has broken a limb before can empathise with you. They have the right receptors activated in their brains to identify with you. They know how you feel, what you are going through, how you might be struggling, what you need, how you will recover. They can empathise with you. It is the ultimate *me too*. Assuming they have a vested interest in you, they lend themselves and their experience to you in a strong display of camaraderie. They will happily tell you what you must do in order to bring your world to order. Then they watch to see if you have followed instructions. If, however, you do not handle your broken leg in as sterling a manner as they did, and your empathiser has a competitive streak, they may adopt a veil of contempt. They sit on their lofty perches and look down on you for being somehow less than they are. Remember the rules, something is bad, apply good corrective measures and return to a state of ordinary bliss. You have been told what to do, you should recover in line with expectation. If you do not, then you must have done something wrong. Black and white.

Sympathy on the other hand is the next rung out on the ripple of responses. They have never had a broken leg, so they have no experience to compare it with. They do care about you though and don't want you to suffer, so they extend sympathy to you in an attempt to make you feel better. There-there, how terrible. Everything will be alright. They may as well sing Soft Kitty (my favourite *Big Bang Theory* reference). They aren't really interested in the details, because they have no open receptors for that information. The odd juicy tid-bit is good for gossiping though, so they will tolerate a certain amount of your narrative before they shut you down. Their enquiries thereafter become polite and are driven by learned behaviour, good manners etc. It is far safer to pretend you are fine in the first place and keep your troubles to yourself. That way there is no pressure on you to recover according to their expectations and no one need patronise you with stupid, useless platitudes.

I know I sound bitter here and perhaps I am, but I speak from experience. I am part of a number of online support groups for chronically ill people. All incredibly brave and wonderful warrior folk who, without exception, feel discounted by their medical supports when they don't respond as expected; or if they have the temerity to suffer from something unidentifiable. Their peer group write them off because they are often forced to cancel arrangements and they become unreliable friends. Their families turn on them as they become a never-ending drain on resources and energy. They go underground. They hide in plain sight. There are hordes and masses of these people.

There is so much that the medical field cannot account for; that science has not yet discovered. People are suffering from disjointed, illogical arrays of symptoms for which there is currently no solution. Once a certain critical mass is achieved, a new syndrome will be named, for example chronic fatigue or fibromyalgia or my personal favourite, atypical-anything or idiopathic-something or other. That just means cause unknown. Patients are given symptom masking drugs that make them more ill. They are passed from pillar to post within the medical profession and they generally end up in the waste basket of the psychiatry department. When nothing else fits, it must be depression. I believe there is something much larger at play here and I remain righteously indignant on behalf of these brave warriors whose lives are for the most part extremely limited.

There is an entire community of Lyme disease sufferers. The medical authorities state categorically that there is no Lyme disease in South Africa, yet I am connected via an online support group with so many people for whom this dreadful condition is their daily reality. In some rare cases, they have laboratory tests to prove it and yet still they cannot be treated. Why? Because officially, it doesn't exist, or their medical practitioners don't know how to treat it. Treatments levied are generally inadequate and cause acute conditions to become chronic. The rest of their lives will be spent searching the world for answers; looking for relief from their daily suffering. They will bankrupt themselves financially, mentally and emotionally as they suffer disappointment after disappointment. Any treatments they do receive, set up a cascade of additional symptoms, as they are poisoned by the toxins created by the die off of the causative bacteria. I pray for you all my Lyme warriors. You are screaming in plain sight and no one is listening to you. There is hope however, as more and more public figures are starting to speak out about their struggle with Lyme disease. People who are world renowned and largely celebrated individuals with enormous reach, not to mention financial reserves… their voices are beginning to be heard. This is a situation that can no longer be denied. Research shows that tick born bacteria was actually weaponised during the second world war. This is a fact that the powers that be have tried to suppress. Almost daily I am seeing new articles on social media that expose this abhorrent truth and it is my greatest wish that the scientists responsible for unleashing this aberration into the world, will turn their considerable talents to the good and will come up with a cure.

I have gone off at a tangent again. I do apologise. On one occasion I had a biopsy done on my tender bits to try and identify the cause of the disgusting rash that had plagued me for years. I'd thrown a bit of a tantrum at the gynae's office when he told me it was a dermatological issue and not for him to deal with. In my experience this is generally code for I don't know. My inner warrior actually made an in-the-flesh appearance as I reminded him that he had been present for the entire curriculum at medical school. As a qualified surgeon he was perfectly capable of doing a biopsy and since it was right on the one part of the body that was most definitely governed by his speciality, he should consider getting his finger out of his arse and bloody well earn the exorbitant fees he was charging. His wasn't a bloody sorting office and I wasn't taking my pants off for anyone else. So, he should just have at it and stop jerking me around! My Dad did warn me about that mouth of mine, but really!!!! Clearly stunned by my vitriol, I was slotted into his already full surgical slate for the next day and the biopsy was performed. Results inconclusively stated that I had dermatitis. Well I bloody well knew that already didn't I. That was why I was there in the first place, because my derma was -itis'd. I took my tube of cortisone cream, accepted that there was nothing to be done and left. Just one more thing to supress and plaster over. Just as well I wasn't open to relationships.

The night of the biopsy, I had tickets to a Queen revue at the theatre. Still anesthetised in the stitched up, tender bits, I donned my jeans and headed for the theatre. It was a group booking made by a friend and I found myself seated next to a most fascinating chap. He was larger than life and his uncontained joy at the revue was something to behold. During the performance, my anaesthetic started to wear off and my tender bits throbbed in time with the rock music, but I didn't care. I was completely mesmerised by this chap. I wanted some of what he had. I wanted to be able to express myself fully and without reserve with not a thought or consideration for anyone else. We went to a pub after the show. I was very uncomfortable in pubs, they smelt like beer and beer fumes triggered all manner of fear and self-loathing in me. On this particular evening though I did not care. I was swept along by this larger than life individual and I felt completely safe with him. We danced, we laughed, we drank and at some point, he picked me up and perched me on his shoulder. I squealed with delight. I was like a toddler at a party.

By the next morning, good sense and order had been restored and I had suffered no ill effects from my adventure. I found in the light of day that I considered him to be a bit of a dodgy individual and I was glad he didn't know how to contact me. I received a phone call from him at the office later that day, saying he had gotten my number from a mutual acquaintance who was at the revue. Together with his fiancé, he owned a Ballroom and Latin American dance studio. He wanted to dance with me and do public demonstrations. He thought we would make a great team. Well who can resist that?

Life Lessons:

- Keep yourself to yourself
- Trust no one

- Be grateful for what you have and protect it for all you're worth
- There is so much suffering in the world
- Evil does exist
- I want to dance

Chapter 19

The Ballroom vs Latin conundrum

Dancing for me, was an absolute revelation. It put me in touch with my body in ways other than simply experiencing pain. Oh, don't get me wrong, there was pain alright, but I knew what was causing it so I could celebrate it. I learned all the Ballroom and Latin American dances and I thrilled to them all. My teacher was a wonderful dancer. He could indicate to me by applying a slight pressure on my back with just one finger, to execute a chasse or, with the heel of his hand to do a lock step. I felt so safe with him. He guided and executed steps and I flowed along with him. We travelled around that floor to the accompanying music and I couldn't have been more thrilled. It wasn't always easy for me. I suffered with joint pain and fatigue and if truth be told, I am not a natural dancer. I have poor balance, doubtful coordination and I was at times, clumsy, obstinate and difficult. I trod on his feet, I hung on his arms, I got frustrated and some days I was a nightmare. But he didn't tell me I was awful or useless or suggest that I should stop for the sake of his feet. He laughed at me and just kept trying to find ways to communicate with my silly body so that it could understand. He would demonstrate the steps with his fiancé and I would wonder how on earth he expected me to pull off such silky-smooth manoeuvres, but somehow, I learned and I loved it.

Ex-Husband came and joined the dance studio. I'll never know quite what prompted him to do so as he had never shown the slightest interest in dancing when we were together. We had never been adversarial divorcees. He had my house keys and he could come and see the girls whenever he wished. He read to the children every night and was as involved in their lives as he wanted to be. He was a fantastic father and my not being able to live with him wasn't something that should cost the girls their father. We even went on the occasional family vacation together. However, when he pitched up at the studio for dance lessons, I was stunned. Before long the children joined as well and we became the equivalent of a modern-day vaudeville act.

The incredible young couple who owned and ran the studio had so much talent and such wonderful ideas. Their business grew organically and they allowed us to showcase our dancing at demonstration evenings, dinner theatre, community carnivals and eventually, on stage at local theatres. Each increase in exposure bought a new layer of learning. There was cutting and editing music, choreography, staging, costume design, dress making, set design, props, stage management, sound, lighting. We knew nothing and we learned as we went along. I'll never forget our first full on production that was open to ticket buying public at a small theatre in town. Studio rehearsals done, costumes done, props done, everything transported to the theatre and we were ready for the off. That dress rehearsal was a dismal flop. Every number was danced on an undressed black stage and we had no lighting. The numbers didn't run together well and there were massive gaps while we rushed to change our costumes. What to do? We could write some sort of jargon about each piece of music, find some singers who wanted to get some exposure to use as fillers, hire a lighting board (and figure out how to use it), get every teenager we knew onboard to man spot lights and… get me to compere the show. I would just prattle on and entertain the audience with interesting snippets about the songs and artists and fill in with witty repartee while the costume changes were happening. I would wind the curtain, operate the lighting board and cue the music. No problem.

I danced the opening number to Elvis Presley's, Jail House Rock. Now remember that I'm a ton overweight and I have lupus; add to that the fact that rock and roll numbers are fast! I led the dash off the stage at the end of the number, snatched up the microphone waiting in the wings and announced in a breathless undertone, "Good evening ladies and gentlemen." Horror of horrors I hadn't managed to catch my breath properly and the resultant sound that came out of me would have made a bad seventies porn star famous. I had no choice but to continue and I compered the entire production sounding like Bambi Woods in *Debbie does Dallas.*

I flickered lights, turned microphones on and off, took care of the singers, changed my costumes in the wings, purred in sultry tones in between to fill any gaps and pulled off my own numbers with only a few mistakes. Thus, we jollied along to the penultimate number. It was a theatre arts piece performed by the studio owners and it contained big scary lifts and huge highlights. We had hired a smoke machine for added drama. I danced off stage at the end of the previous number, cued their music, slid down onto the floor, located the right button in the dark and as the music started to play, I pressed the button on the smoke machine. It was facing the wrong way and I completely gassed myself. I whipped it around to face the stage and then almost had a convulsion trying not to cough during their big number. Then up again I jumped and danced the finale to Will Young's, *Evergreen*. My goodness, what an experience. We couldn't wait to start planning the next production.

With each show, we got better. Anything that went wrong in a production was ironed out by the next one. We were learning and we were loving it. The growth of these two individuals was a joy to behold and they generously dragged all of us along in their wake. We were an amateur social dance studio and our cast of characters was made up of people from seven to seventy, the fit and the fat, the talented and the rest of us, the dancers and the wannabes, the beginners and the more accomplished. It made no difference. Each student was encouraged to live out their dreams and fantasies and numbers were choreographed to show them off in the best possible light. Costumes were designed to thrill and delight and we had a blast. While we were largely short on talent, we were high on energy and enthusiasm. Somehow that translated to the audiences. For one particularly lovely production I had gone on radio and promoted ticket sales. We were not great at the marketing side, but for this one we had a solution. We had programmes designed and we had that radio slot. That was the only show where we received a complaint from an audience member who said, he found it offensive that he had paid good money to see a dancing show and he was forced to watch fat people waddling around on stage. Well, we understood that there's one in every crowd, so we gave him back his money and as a chorus we shouted, "Well fuck you too!"

The decade spent dancing with these wonderful souls gave me some of the best times of my life. In a theatre environment, I didn't want to hide, oh no! I wanted the spotlight, the microphone, the centre stage. I thrilled standing on a stage in the glare of the lights, holding the audience in the palm of my hand. I could make them laugh and I could still them with a word. I could whip them into an evangelical frenzy with just the right tone of voice… and I loved it! I have learned through my studies of weird shit, that music is one of the greatest gifts given to human beings. It is designed to bring us into the light. It has a purity and intensity that can lift even the most maudlin of people up and turn them into happy, empowered beings. I had been right all those years ago in church when I decided that music was where all the joy in the world emanated from. I'm forever grateful to my teachers for being allowed, nay encouraged, to shine. For being celebrated no matter the quality of the output. For being made to feel that I mattered, that I had something to contribute and most importantly, that I belonged. They will never fully know the extent of the gifts they gave each of their students. My prayer is that that joy is returned to them a thousand-fold, for it is only as they deserve.

Life Lessons:

- The family that plays together, stays together
- Be prepared to take risks
- With the right encouragement you can do anything
- Always find a great teacher when tackling a new skill
- I love the spotlight!

Chapter 20

The win a few, lose a few conundrum

My magnificent horse, the love of my life, had a problem. He would be fine one minute and completely lame the next. I remember the day the vet came to examine him. He asked me to trot him up and down so he could observe his movements. The vet called to me as I trotted away. I stopped the horse and twisted around to talk to him. I placed my hand on my horse's rump behind me as I turned… well I would have done if he hadn't swung out sideways. I fell hard and broke my wrist. I wonder how many other people have broken a wrist while standing completely still on a horse. The horse was diagnosed as having kissing spines. Cliff note version:

Kissing spines refers to a condition in horses in which two or more of the spinous processes (the flanges of bone sticking up from each vertebra in the spine) are positioned so that they touch or rub against each other. Horse with kissing spines may develop back pain, bone cysts, arthritic changes, and other problems.

I turned my horse out to rest as there wasn't anything to be done. I couldn't bear for him to be in pain and so riding was out of the question. I was introduced to a retired army chap who had a great space that he rented out for horses such as mine to retire to. Our relationship became one of carrots, cuddles and communion. Unfortunately, he caught a very bad dose of Spanish horse flu that was ripping through stable yards all over town and he never came back to full health. I had to make the decision to let him go. The vet refused to euthanise him if I was present and I will always regret not being there for his final moments. It is such a privilege to be paired with a horse. They are one of the most incredible creatures on this green earth and the relationship one has with them is, in my opinion, unparalleled. I would find out more about that in years to come. For now though, my heart was broken.

Many years later I attended a vision board workshop. It was run by an ex colleague of mine who had quit the corporate world to follow her passion as a psychic medium. She had done the same courses I had, but she grabbed it with both hands and dived in. I saw her once for a reading and my take home from it was, "Be careful of climbing the ladder of success, only to find it is leaning up against the wrong wall." Anyhow, she was running the workshop and I was curious to see what it entailed. We spent the entire morning paging through magazines of all shapes and sizes. The instruction was to tear out anything that caught our eye, pictures, words, headlines, colour... anything at all. We were instructed not to think about it too much and to just let rip. We broke for lunch and then we went back in and sorted through the pile of clippings. It was so interesting to see how similar so many of them were. When they were all grouped together, it became apparent that there were six identifiable topics in front of me. We then created collages and stuck everything onto a board. The premise here is that your unconscious mind will guide you and you will tear out things related to your heart's desires. Some of those desires, you may not even be consciously aware of. Mine related primarily to health, strength, hope, good nutrition, writing and right up front and centre, Mauritius. That last one surprised me.

Fast forward a while and the office have launched a staff incentive. There were goals, objectives and targets and the winner would get an all-expenses paid trip to Mauritius. That caught my attention. I had been listening to some tapes on the subject of manifestation and positive thinking and I decided to set my sights on the Mauritius trip. Please understand I was way down on the workplace food chain and the chances of my winning that trip were – well, not very good. I didn't care about that though, I acted as though I had already won it. I told everyone I met that the office was sending me to Mauritius. I updated my passport and that was that, I was going. Come the day of the grand reveal and I was still telling everyone that I was so excited to be going to Mauritius. The winner's name was read out and it wasn't mine. I wobbled for a few seconds, but then remembered what I had learned about manifesting and I immediately started thinking of other ways to get myself there. I was going to Mauritius if it was the last thing I did. I realised that everyone was oohing and aahing and I decided I should pay attention. The directors had been so impressed with the response to their goal setting exercises that they had decided to award an additional nine winners for the Mauritius trip and we would go together as a group. It was everything I dreamed it would be and so much more.

Life Lessons:

- Do your duty for your loved ones, no matter how much it hurts
- Nothing lasts forever
- Dare to dream
- Don't take no for an answer
- Mama likes to travel

Chapter 21

The home isn't home anymore conundrum

My daughters were grown by now and were ready to leave the nest. At twenty-one and eighteen they wanted to head off to England and have an adventure. The one good thing I have done for my children is I was British born. They had EU passports and had a much freer access to international travel than their South African counterparts. I am forgiven many transgressions in the name of the EU passport. I have invoked its power to save myself on more than one occasion when I was being blamed for something that I had purportedly done to ruin their lives. Even the best kids go through a stage where they find their parents inadequate and disappointing. Thank goodness this generally doesn't last.

My eldest arranged herself a job and accommodation for both of them with mutual friends they had met during their summer jobs. The youngest would pound pavements on arrival and find herself some work. They booked their flights and the dreaded day came when we took them to the airport. I wanted them to leave feeling excited and fired up. I would be brave and I would shield them from my churning emotions. These girls were the one good thing I had ever done in my life and without them I had no idea who I was or what my purpose in life would be. However, I was confident I had raised them well and as they set off to face the unknown, they were brave and bold and beautiful and I was so proud. I stayed strong for them as I waved them goodbye. I left the airport and I have no idea how I drove because I felt like I was outside of my body. I drove to a shopping mall, crawled into the back row of a movie theatre and sobbed through the same movie (don't ask me what it was about) three times before I felt able to face the world again.

When I arrived home, I was met by a very depressed little sausage dog. My daughter's dog would stay with me while she travelled. His sad little face gave me a focus for my feelings and I held him tight as we both adjusted to our new, strange, quiet home that didn't feel like home anymore. My Great Dane was unperturbed. He was one hundred percent my dog and I was the epicentre of his universe. As long as we were together, he was one happy fellow. He climbed onto my bed and lay along the length of my back and it almost felt as though he was shoring up my spine, giving me the added strength that I needed to handle this painful, if inevitable transition. Sausages are noisy little buggers and the quiet component of life was quickly shattered as he adjusted, his depression lifted and he got on with the business of being a happy little sausage.

My Great Dane had come to me quite out of the blue. A friend had sent me an email to show me the sweet little Great Dane pup she was getting. I didn't even see him to be honest. My eyes locked onto the black pup sitting on the grass behind him and I just knew he had to be mine. He was promised to someone else, but I didn't care. And mine, he most certainly was. The breeder drove the two pups down to where we stayed and I went to my friend's house to meet my guy. She opened the back of her car and this little love bug climbed up my body, put a paw on either side of my neck and snuggled in for a hug. That pretty much sums up our entire relationship. He was my second great love.

With an enormous gaping hole in my life caused by the departure of my children, I was completely at sea. I needed to be occupied, I needed a new challenge. When the office moved to a new plant they had built and they were looking for a facilities manager, I volunteered my services. I was most surprised when they accepted. I don't even change my own light bulbs at home, I hire a handy man, but they didn't know that. What in the world was I thinking? I was right out of my comfort zone, but that was good because I was completely focussed on my new job requirements and I had no time to think about my aching heart. I learned to commission a generator, operate the electric fences, manually override a stuck lift, program the computers to water the gardens, read plans and so many other things I had never even thought about. We moved into a building site with a snag list as long as the Nile River, builders swarming everywhere and just a tad of chaos. Cement was dropped down the lift shaft onto the front of someone's brand new car on my first day in. I sent the hysterical chap upstairs to work and assured him his car would be sorted by the end of the day. How? No clue, but I found out and when he came down at the end of the day ready for battle, I was one smug, self-satisfied bunny as I handed him the keys to his immaculately clean, unscathed vehicle.

A million bits of information floated all over the place and knowledge lived in people's heads. I knew from previous experience how undesirable that is. People should leave work at the end of the day with clear heads so that they can focus on their home lives and be where they are at. Trying to store a million bits of information in your brain just leads to burnout and… well frankly, loss of information. I set to work and built an intranet site and I loaded every piece of information I could find, from the building plans right down to the phone number for the locksmith who had cut our spare keys, and GPS coordinates for the paint shop where we bought our paint, along with the paint colour references of course. Anything I didn't know how to do, I created a How-To Manual and loaded it onto the intranet. By the time I was finished, anyone could have accessed any piece of information regarding that building and our campus was, facilities-wise, fully documented. I had successfully worked myself out of a job.

A challenge of the unexpected kind came one morning when there was a baby snake in the downstairs basement parking garage. I called for one of the security guards to bring me a box and he arrived with a paper wrapper from a batch of photocopy paper. We were starting to attract a crowd and I wanted this dealt with, so I grabbed the packet and managed to coax the feisty little bugger into the bag. Well pleased with myself I rolled the top over and proceeded to walk through the office reception to go and release it into the garden. I hadn't realised there was a tear in the packet until the little guy stuck his head out and hissed at me. That was the day I broke the world record for fastest sprint.

I spent a lot of time at the office. It became my home away from home. I preferred to be there than in my quiet house. Often, I was there on weekends and evenings. There was always more work to be done and I was more than happy to do it. I would often take my Great Dane with me for company. The security guards weren't too keen on my giant black dog, but that wasn't my problem. One night my phone rang at 3am. It was the security guards on the phone. There was an intruder in the office and I was to please bring the big black dog and come and rescue them. Security guards on night duty in this country are not a very educated, well paid, well trained lot and nothing was worth them getting hurt. They knew if they phoned their control room they would have been forced to investigate and it made far more sense to call the boss lady with the big black dog to check it out for them. I loaded my trusty boy into the car and we raced round to the office. Now they had a conundrum of their own. They had to show me where they had seen the intruder, but that entailed them coming out of the guard house and communing with the big grinning dog. With a little encouragement from me, tactfully and respectfully delivered, you understand, we were on our way to go and flush out the bad guys. The guards hid themselves like scared little boys behind a low wall and pointed in the general direction of the CFOs office. There glowing in the moonlight was the bronze bust of Nelson Mandela that had been delivered to him recently. It had pride of place on his window ledge awaiting its final location to be decided.

Life Lessons:

- Sometimes your success at a job is measured by your ability to work yourself out of that job (motherhood, facilities management)
- A mother's heart can tear in two and she can still stay alive
- You can have more than one great love in your life
- Baby snakes are more venomous than their adult versions
- Scooby Doo rides again

Chapter 22

The down under conundrum

Travelling became another area of life where I knew the joy was stored. By now the list was growing. I had found joy in singing (sadly the long years of coughing without respite had rendered my vocals rough and limited in range, so that was over); horses (that was over now too. I never rode again after I lost my horse); energy work (I had shut that down because I was a coward); music and dancing (the studio closed down when the couple split up and after a long ten year run, that too was over); of course, my children (although they had left home by now as well); and now I have found travel. Travel cost money though, money I didn't have. When an ex colleague, with whom I had become close friends during our Mauritius trip, emigrated to Australia and invited another friend and I to visit her, I maxed out every credit card I had and I hopped that plane. There are some joys that simply should not be denied.

We had a magnificent holiday. Our friends made us feel so welcome and they spoiled us from the moment we landed until we left, sobbing, three weeks later. My friend's young son was our tour guide and he provided facts and information that fascinated and sometimes horrified us. Australia isn't a gentle country and he delighted in telling us about various nightmares of nature like poisonous snakes and Huntsmen spiders that were the size of dinner plates and could only be killed by blowing hot air on them. We looked around for the cowboy style holsters loaded with cordless hair driers that we clearly needed to survive in this place, but to no avail. We took him at his word in every situation, although he could have been talking utter rubbish, we guzzled it all up. We were so grateful for his vast knowledge and selflessness and for that extra special element he added to our trip. Sydney is an incredibly beautiful city and we must have taken thousands of photographs. We had the time of our lives.

Every day we went out exploring and there were so many highlights I could almost write an entire book about the trip, but there were three things that stood out for me where I learned the greatest lessons. Firstly, I learned that true friends are a source of joy. True friends accept you as is, warts and all and they love you in spite of yourself. They are few and far between and they are precious beyond rubies. They are not high maintenance relationships and they grow organically. They want only the best for you and they find and nurture the best in you. They do not judge you and they support you without question. These were such friends and I remain forever grateful for having them be a part of my life.

The second thing I learned is that laughter truly is the best medicine. I had taken a lot of strain on the long seventeen-hour flight. I had the passenger in front of me, seat fully reclined, lying in my lap all the way. I had requested the flight attendant to ask them to please sit up when breakfast was served, but apparently it is their policy not to disturb passengers sleeping behind eye masks. My inner child screamed inside my head, "Well fuck you too!" at the hostess. As she turned away, I pulled hard on the woman's hair. I quickly lay back and closed my eyes (talk about a child!). She mumbled and muttered and was clearly annoyed at having been woken up after only sleeping for twelve hours, poor dear, but since I had been cradling her stupid head in my lap, unable to move the entire time, I couldn't have cared less.

She went to the toilet and I slipped into her seat and raised it upright. Anyhow, I digress again. My feet and legs were very swollen when we arrived in Australia, exhausted but excited. There was no definition from toes to knees, my legs looked like blown up balloons and they hurt. I had been in hospital just prior to leaving for our trip with an asthma attack that went on for ten days. My doctor had suggested I not fly. Well that wasn't going to happen, so he gave me some self-injectable stuff to prevent blood clots that I had to administer in the airport bathroom just before boarding, and he reluctantly agreed I could go. I wasn't feeling great when we arrived, but excitement was the order of the day and all health problems were firmly shoved aside. I would take part in everything even if it killed me. I wouldn't be the handbrake on this holiday.

We went out one day on a jetboating experience. We climbed into the purple rain gear provided, strapped ourselves into the seats of this speed boat and waited to see what it was all about. The driver roared that boat around the Sydney Harbour at speeds that were utterly ridiculous, it felt incredibly dangerous and yet thrilling at the same time. At a moment's notice he would throw the craft into a three hundred and sixty degree turn that threw us on top of one another and had us all drenched in spray as we drove through our own wake. The shrieking and laughing that went down on that boat was something I shall never forget. As we were thrown this way and that way, soaking spray and churning stomachs, we laughed fit to bust. We laughed until our bellies and our faces hurt. I climbed off that boat at the end feeling younger and lighter than I had in years.

The third thing I learned is that I truly, am my own worst enemy. Mother was a woman afraid of most things and she practiced absolute avoidance at all costs. I was determined that I would never let fear be a reason not to do something and I was keen to try everything that came my way. I didn't necessarily seek out dangerous or challenging situations, but if ever I found myself struggling with the heat of the kitchen, I didn't get out as the saying goes; no, I grabbed a sauté pan and I cooked the shit out it. For anyone who is wondering, since I'm claiming to be all feel the fear and do it anyway how come I quit the rehab? Well, fear and cowardice are two very different things. Fear is defined as an unpleasant emotion caused by the threat of danger, pain, or harm. Cowardice is a lack of bravery. This is why in spite of being very afraid of heights, I climbed that Sydney Harbour Bridge and I posed at the tippy tippy top for photographs to prove it. I sobbed all the way up the sheer sides of the tower building, almost paralysed with fear; skipped over the top of the bridge part quite comfortably since it was stairs all the way; and nearly had heart failure on the way down the opposite tower. My friend cried too and her husband said following the two of us was like herding wet cats.

Life Lessons:

- When people love and accept you, let them
- It is acceptable to fly now and pay later provided you can handle the debt
- I have rights too, dammit!
- Nothing good ever happens in your comfort zone
- Laughter is the best medicine
- Feel the fear and do it anyway
- I am brave, but sometimes it's prudent to just stay out of the kitchen altogether

Chapter 23

The Humpty Dumpty conundrum

I was attending the wedding of a good friend. My entire family were part of the retinue and it was a lavish affair. We were dressed up in our Italian designer gowns, hair coiffed and make-up expertly applied. Everything was going beautifully. The bride's two-year-old was being a little fractious during the long photography session. She was demanding that we take her home immediately and mom had to come too. I muttered at her to stop being such a little nut-job. Well that was the wrong thing to do because she shrieked, "Nut job, nut job," at the top of her considerable little voice throughout the rest of the photographs. Oops! Sorry.

The bride and groom went off for their private photographs while the rest of us enjoyed canapes and cocktails and watched a polo match. At the end of the match, the polo players raced to one end of the field and took up a formation with mallets held aloft and the club's anthem was played over loudspeakers. The anthem was probably the most stirring piece of music I had ever heard and I immediately felt as though I had gone to war and lost everyone I loved and that the world as I knew it was ending. I was gripped by a deep soul sadness that left me feeling gutted and sobbing. I wasn't the only one it seemed, and when the poor bride climbed out of the Rolls Royce, which the polo payers has escorted down the field, instead of a joy filled welcome, she found half her guests in tears. It was certainly dramatic.

The rest of the wedding went off without a hitch with one small exception. As I stepped down from the veranda onto the gravelled path below, my shoe broke and I fell. The big toe on my right foot bent right over backwards and the pain was unimaginable. Ex-Husband hauled me to my feet and wincing with pain, I limped to the bathroom. We agreed the toe looked shocking. I was in agony, but I wasn't going to spoil the bride's evening and miss all the fun. I rammed my foot into the leather pumps I had in my bag for emergencies (this definitely qualified), took two paracetamol and smiled and waved my way through the reception.

The next morning, we were going away with other friends for our annual get away from it all vacation. These guys had a share in a farm four hour's drive away. There was dust road access and it was positioned on a river about fourteen kilometres outside of a small seaside town on a winding, bone rattling, dangerous road. We had no electricity or mobile phone signal and amenities were rugged at best. We had some incredible times there together. The bunkrooms where we were sleeping were at the top of a rough-cut natural stone staircase and the loo was outside around the other side of the bunk room. My foot was throbbing and I was a little unsteady, but I wasn't going to fuss and spoil everyone's holiday. Well that was the plan anyway.

At 3am I was dying to go to the loo, so I shuffled out of my sleeping bag and into my slippers yelping, "Ow!" as my poor sprained foot protested. Treading gingerly, I stepped down onto the path. My foot gave way and I stumbled. I had no way of saving myself as I stumbled at an ever-increasing speed, two or three paces and with my head thrust forward, I dived over the edge. I flew down a four-meter drop and landed upside down, breaking my fall by smashing the top of my head into the side of the house. I was twisted like a pretzel and I thought I had broken my neck. I couldn't move, I couldn't even identify which limb was which. My neck was twisted one way and my back in the other direction. I called out for help and the noise that came out of me was utterly primal. I was shocked by the sound I was making. It didn't sound like me at all, but more like a cornered terrified animal.

I broke the big toes on both feet, tore the muscles along my sternum, and concussed myself. I didn't know it at the time, but I had also broken my back. A bed was set up in the lounge and I was given an anti-inflammatory injection (ex-Husband had his doctor's bag) and was settled as comfortably as possible for the rest of the night. I had upset a lot of people, children included, and everyone was on edge. Ex-Husband slept on the couch to watch over me. Anxious to save the situation I declared I was fine to stay on and everyone should carry on with their holiday I would just lie in the bed and stay out of the way. My girls were incredible and they helped me to perform the basics of toileting and hair washing. I was unable to do anything for myself. Five days later, I was carefully packed into the car and we left for home. Tackling the rough dust road was a challenge.

The day after arriving back in town, I went to my GP to get the once over. He was going on holiday the next day, but he assured me that my injuries were pretty serious and he would be sure to phone me with the results and an action plan before he left. He didn't. I never went back to him again. I was his patient, something massively traumatic had happened to me, I was broken and in pain and he couldn't be arsed to call me back.

I did the best I could, but I confess I rushed my recovery. The doctor was clearly not bothered, so I assumed it wasn't serious and I just got on with it. In the early days, if I needed to turn over in bed at night, I would have to phone one of my girls sleeping in their rooms across the passage, to come and help me. I was in a right state. Friends were great and helped me to get to appointments with my wonderful chiropractor. I trusted him completely and he saw me every second day for the first two weeks. Then once I was back at work, we stretched it out little by little over the next six months until I was seeing him monthly. Did I care for myself properly? No. I was expected back at the office, plus I hated to be dependent on anyone for help, so as soon as I could think straight (which I took to mean the concussion had resolved), I mashed my sore feet into some half way functional slippers and dived right in. I still struggle with allowing anyone to help me.

Life Lessons:

- Don't mess with a two-year-old
- Sometimes you should put yourself first
- Demand proper care and accept nothing less
- My girls are amazing
- I am not important enough to be treated right

Chapter 24

The Dubai conundrum

Fast track three years and I'm feeling terrible. I had so much pain in my body, some days I battled to breathe. I struggled with sleep and there were periods of up to ten days at a time where I never closed my eyes. I had asthma, violent migraine headaches, I trembled, sweated and shook, and I felt like hell. My feet burned all the time and I couldn't bear to have closed shoes on.

At this time, I was running an online shopping mall for my company and I had a team working under me. I was going on out of town business trips to see suppliers and visit trade shows, I was doing product selections, quality checking all of my team's product loading work, copywriting, handling the HR component of the department, as well as strategic and tactical planning, reporting, client interactions and promotional calendars, plus I was part of the team managing the staff incentive scheme. I had so much work on my plate, I rarely left before 9 or 10pm. People were in and out of my office all day long asking me questions, what to do, how to do it, help me with this, help me with that, please join a meeting. On and on it went in an ever faster spinning merry go round. Once the staff had gone home, I would begin my day and tackle my to do list. Madness! Come time to compute the results of the staff incentive program however, I am the company's top performer for the year. I am thrilled as this means I've won a trip to Dubai.

For the third year in a row I end up in hospital with a two-week long asthma attack. The doctors nebulise and medicate me and warn me to take things easy. They tell me I have chronic obstructive airway disease and will need medication for the rest of my life. Once again, I am handed a life-limiting diagnosis. I think about it long and hard and realise that since I only suffer seasonally from these asthma attacks and for the rest of the year, I manage just fine, this cannot be the case. This time I reject the diagnosis. I will find a way to deal with the seasonal allergies and I will not spend another spring or autumn in hospital… and I never have. My doctors advised me most strenuously against travelling so soon after being hospitalised, but what the hell do they know?

Dubai was incredible. I had no preconceived ideas about it and I was thrilled and delighted with everything we did and saw there. The group was going to Ferrari World for the day and my friend and I were not keen. We booked instead to go hot air ballooning over the desert at sunrise. Now, I don't do mornings. There were days that I wandered around the office faking being awake and pretending I was actually alive until sometime, usually at around 10 or 11am, when the fog in my brain would lift, my pulse would kick in and I would be fully all there. Anything before then was a bit of a blur. I had been a reluctant starter my whole life, but it had definitely become more of a challenge with each passing year.

At 4 a.m. we were collected at reception by our German pilot, who I estimated to be about 6'8". I have never met such a tall man. We arrived at the launch sight and found, what we learned, was the largest hot air balloon in the world, lying flat on the sand. The crew were preparing it for the launch. Dubai is extreme like that, whatever is to be found in the West, they emulate, but theirs is slightly bigger, longer, taller, faster and somehow elevated. We peered into the pre-dawn dark and watched this monster balloon slowly begin to inflate. The pilot came over and announced in a large, booming, German-accented voice, "When balloon is up, and I say run, you run! Balloon is up, she must go, so you hurry." Got it. Clear instructions. Race across the sand and hop into the basket. Easy.

Next minute he started to bellow, "Run, run!!" Well I ran and the closer I got to the balloon, the clearer it became that the basket was, in fact, almost chest height. How the hell would I be able to heave my huge, 100 kg plus bulk up into it. Well, apparently, all that is required to draw immense athletic ability from me is a screaming 6'8" pilot and the dread of missing out. I placed my hand on the top rail and vaulted, just like a gymnast, neatly into the basket. My stunned friend (that made two of us), gasped, "Get out and do that again, I need that on video." She had climbed in using the cut-out foot holds in the side of the basket that I hadn't even noticed in my mad dash.

The trip was a true life's highlight and I am so grateful we could share this amazing experience. We weren't quite done yet though. When landing, we had to stand with our backs facing the direction we were going with our knees slightly bent, holding on tight to the railings and braced. The basket hit the ground at one hell of a speed and it bounced a few times and swayed as it was dragged along in the sand by the still full balloon. Eventually we came to a stop which was great, except that we were suspended about three feet in the air having held onto the centre part of the balloon. There was nothing for it, but to launch ourselves out of the balloon in a backward somersault, landing on the sand. The dismount definitely cost me the gold medal.

Another great memory I have is from the day we went dune bashing in 4X4 vehicles. I felt horrendously car sick the entire time, but I had begged my way into the front seat, so I knew I could open a window and not vomit on anyone and if the worst came to the worst I would throw myself from the vehicle (dramatic much!) Well I didn't need to do any of that and we had a most thrilling time driving up the steep dunes and then sliding precariously down again. My inner hooligan was happy. We sat on the hot sand and watched the sun go down in one of the most spectacular settings. It was quite awe inspiring in spite of me feeling green around the gills. Next, we were taken to a Bedouin village and were treated to henna tattoos, whirling dervish dancing and so much more. We ended the evening with a glorious feast. None of this was helping my pallor to recover so I grabbed one of my colleagues and said, "Let's go and do something to shake my ears right so I can enjoy the evening. "Seems logical, I feel like crap, go and do something extreme to refocus your mind.

We found the camel riding guys. She hopped up nimbly onto her camel, but I wasn't so sure I had another athletic feat in me. Next moment one of the chaps came running with a large white bucket shouting, "I bring bucket for big lady to get onto camel. Camel very strong, can take three men. Perhaps big lady plus one more." At that point my colleague nearly fell off her camel laughing. Red in the face and smarting with embarrassment I gingerly mounted the camel from my bucket, listening closely for sounds of groaning from the beast. He seems to be fine and praying he wouldn't collapse under me, I held on tight as he lurched to his feet, slamming the pommel of the saddle into my solar plexus and knocking the wind right out of me. Well that definitely took care of my ears, I had more important things to focus on now, like breathing. After riding a thoroughbred horse for years, I found riding a camel to be a bizarre experience. It feels as though they walk one leg at a time and their gait is ungainly and uncomfortable. However, we travelled around the village and I kept all such treasonous thoughts to myself, not wanting to offend my camel in any way lest he keel over. Getting back to where we started, there was no bucket for big lady to get off the camel and once again, I had to resort to throwing myself off sideways into the sand. What is it with this place and the wretched dismount?

Life Lessons:

- No matter how bad your feel, get up, dress up, and show up, fake it if necessary
- Doctors are useless to me
- I am a closet gymnast
- Camels are very strong

Chapter 25

The apnoea conundrum

I had shared a room with my friend on the Dubai trip. She spent most of the night prodding me and poking me to get me to stop snoring. All she did was make bruises and we ended up trading rooms. My new bunk mate took sleeping tablets and couldn't care less what noise I made, so we were sorted. My friend lobbied the idea of sleep apnoea at me. Now if you remember I did have a sleep study done previously, after my first child was born, but it hadn't shown any problems. Rather shocked at how much of an issue my snoring had been, I decided to have a repeat study done. I read up on sleep apnoea and wondered if it wasn't the cause of the bone crushing exhaustion I was feeling. I reported to the sleep lab at the appointed time, had some clips and wires glued to my head and was told to tuck in for the night and go to sleep. I don't know about you, but in a strange environment, wired up like Frankenstein's monster, I'm afraid I found sleep to be elusive. I must have gone off at some point though because I was shaken awake and told I could go home. They would contact me with the results.

Turns out I stop breathing up to twenty-three times an hour. That's almost every two minutes! Then I snort and snore to kick start my engines and off I go again. No wonder I was exhausted. I hadn't had a proper night's sleep in years. I was to come back to the lab to test drive a CPAP mask. I wasn't overly enthused by this idea, (remember I suffer from claustrophobia), but I packed my biggest pair of big girl panties in and presented myself as instructed. Pyjamas on and teeth brushed; the dreaded mask was brought in. Wide eyed and fighting a rising panic, I was fitted with the mask. It covered my nose and mouth and was attached by an elasticated headgear. It had a long flexible pipe that went from the front of the mask to the machine. I was instructed not to breathe through my mouth at all as it would cause a sucking effect. Lots of people were uncomfortable in the beginning I was assured, but since it was the only solution for my problem, I would just have to brace myself and get used to it.

Alrighty then. That was a pretty clear instruction delivered in a snippy tone that brooked no argument, so I lay down, feeling rather sorry for myself and tried to control my rapidly beating heart. The lights were turned out and that was that. No one came near me for the rest of the night. Of course I opened my mouth and the wretched mask sucked itself onto my face like a murderous octopus. I was not a happy camper. At about 3 a.m. I'd had enough. I ripped the mask off and threw it across the room. I sat there sobbing and shaking and wondering how my life had come down to this. All alone in a strange place, terrified and no way out. I looked around for a technician and couldn't find one, so I got dressed and went home. I had a shower and went to the office. Nice early start at 5 a.m., get at a jump on the day.

I was in a state of shock I think, traumatised by the events of the night. I felt backed into a corner and I had no idea how to fight my way out. If I wanted to live long and prosper, I needed to sleep. In order to sleep, I needed to wear the dreaded CPAP. The thought of spending my resting hours tethered to that creature from the deep, while it sucked the life force out of me was more than I could bear. I almost made it right through the day before I began to unravel. One of my staff came in and asked if I was alright, he was concerned about me. That one tiny ounce of kindness was all it took and the dam broke. I grabbed my things, jumped in my car and raced down to a deserted stretch of beach. I did not want to live anymore if living included that evil mask. I felt so ill, I couldn't get help for what ailed me except in this one situation and I couldn't tolerate the solution. I was determined to walk into the sea and let myself be swallowed up by the waves. I was tired. I had been fighting a war on so many fronts my entire life and I felt as though I was fresh out of options. Perhaps it was time to finish it once and for all. I sat there a good long while thinking in swirling circles of misery and despair. Could I find any other solution?

Well I didn't get to find out. My mobile phone rang. One of my daughter's friends, had felt my distress and she was calling to see if I was alright. Another friend had received a call at the office from her daughter asking if she knew why I was sitting all alone on a deserted road next to the sea. I guess I too am not wanted by heaven. I went home and had a total breakdown. I climbed into bed and I wailed and I moaned and I rocked and I reeled and all I could say was, "You'll miss me when I'm gone."

In my darkest hour, I find a modicum of my worth, my worthiness that seems invisible to those around me. Anyone who tried to help me that day, was treated really badly and for that I will always be sorry, but I wasn't in my right mind and honestly, they simply didn't know how to help me in the way that I needed to be helped. All I really needed was for someone to hold me, to connect with me, so that I knew I wasn't completely alone. How could they know what I needed? No one really knew who I was, or what I was going through. And that's on me, because I have hidden in plain sight all of my life.

I did get a CPAP mask in the end, a smaller, less intrusive design that I named Squiddy, given that it was a miniature version of the dreaded octopus. I really did try, but after three months of waking up screaming and sweating in the middle of the night, in the throes of ripping the blasted Squiddy off my face, I called it quits. No one can live in a full-blown panic attack for three months without some serious damage being done. I consulted an endocrinologist, following a hunch and was diagnosed with adrenal insufficiency. She seemed more perturbed by my weight issues however and we ended up parting company when her treatment didn't help me. She changed tactics and proceeded to convince me I was diabetic, even though my blood sugars tested within normal range. Another doctor determined to fit me into the field of her learning and to label me with a life-limiting condition. She simply would not hear me when I protested that I felt no better. How dare I have the temerity to not recover in line with expectations.

Life Lessons:

- Empathy and tact should be taught to anyone dealing with patient care
- If a zookeeper hears hoofbeats, he thinks zebra, even in the absence of stripes
- I need to keep getting up, dressing up and showing up
- Heaven doesn't want me

Chapter 26

The retrenchment conundrum

Life can be so strange. On one hand, I was becoming quite a powerful woman in my own right, whilst at the same time, I felt as though I was fading away physically (all the while becoming more and more overweight). At the end of this story, I think you'll understand, as I eventually did, the psychic's comment to me about the ladder of success leaning against the wrong wall. I had taken a completely left turn in my life. I had abandoned the weird shit entirely and was moving further and further away from my true centre, all the while faking success. It is no wonder I was getting into such a state. Well, I was about to receive a harsh correction.

I was called into the boss's office one day and notified that the company was restructuring and I needed to retrench a certain number of people. I would then absorb another department and essentially do more work with a reduced staff compliment. I was shocked. I could only posit that after this was done, the remaining staff would be left feeling insecure and as a result, unproductive. I wondered how I was meant to pull this all off. However, I had faith in the powers that be, they all had fancy educations after all, and I deferred to their superior knowledge in such matters.

It is not unheard of for corporates to restructure from time to time, and the trimming of resources is a part of that process. Whole teams would be disbanded and everyone would be invited to reapply for their jobs, but only a select number of applicants would be successful as the number of jobs would have been reduced. Neat and tidy, no muss, no fuss. The re-employed, I was assured, would actually feel grateful for their reprieve. Feeling valued for having been selected to stay, they would rise to new heights and tackle the added workload like champions. Duly reassured, I pulled on my corporate big girl loyalty pants and starting moving chess pieces around.

I was already working ridiculous hours and was struggling to stay afloat. My health was appalling and I had developed a new symptom, aphasia. I kept forgetting words. Names were beyond me and I resorted to calling everyone Sweetie or Darling which is so friggin' patronising, I'm still astounded it didn't land me in trouble with HR. I became verbose, because whilst I had no trouble describing in great detail what a kettle was, I simply could not dredge up the actual word. My stress levels rose exponentially with my struggle to speak properly, coupled with my difficulty in focussing and staying awake. The tinnitus in my ears buzzed so loudly it felt as though I had a swarm of angry high-pitched bees trapped inside my brain. I was in hell. But I had a job to do and so I set about planning how to redistribute the workload. The day the letters went out to the affected staff notifying them of the impending retrenchments, I was stunned to see my name was on the list too. The manager of the other department to be disbanded and merged with my team was not included, but there my name sat in black and white. The world turned upside down as I suddenly realised the implications of what I was about to do.

I had a great relationship with my team, they worked hard and did a good job; and they were all lovely people. I would be putting some of them out of work, not because of anything they had done wrong, but because the game was being reset. Thank you for your years of loyalty and sterling effort; you are the weakest link, goodbye. I knew they had children or families to support. Many of them were struggling with their finances already. Some of them were the main breadwinners in their families.

My job was to throw a grenade into their lives. I simply could not do it. This wasn't my dream, this wasn't my business, I was but a small, apparently dispensable cog in someone else's game. I didn't want to be the one to deliver such news to people who had only ever given me of their best efforts. My soul could not deal with that. Plus, there was no guarantee I would even be given my job back if I reapplied. There were younger people coming down the track, with equal if not superior skills, proper education, and they were not ill, faking being alive for most of the day.

I agonised over this situation, I tried out myriad different scenarios in my mind, trying to save as many of them as I could. I became so stressed and tense I actually pinched a nerve in my neck and my entire right arm became a new source of high-level agony. Sleep was out of the question. My mind raced around and around. My team looked to me for guidance and support and I had to betray them. I was standing in the bathroom one day, battling to breathe, staring at myself in the mirror, wondering how everything had gone so horribly wrong, when I heard a voice say, "So what do you want?"

I told the bosses that, in line with my legal rights apropos this situation they had created, I wouldn't be reapplying for my job. I felt that the ask was too big and with my health in the state it was in, I didn't have anything more to give. All hell broke loose. Some very ugly things were said, some unforgivable and completely untrue accusations were levied and I wondered how it was that my loyalty for over two decades had come down to this… naught.

There is no sentiment in business and as with the Jewish mother in law all those years ago, the reality was this had nothing to do with me personally. But from my vantage point, it was another betrayal of the highest order. I had given my best, my all, and I wasn't worthy. It felt pretty bloody personal to me. The CEO who had recognised me all those years before, came to my rescue and called off the attack. I was paid out a very fair retrenchment package and was allowed to leave with as much dignity as I could muster.

I remain, in my heart, forever loyal to him and forever grateful for the learning experiences and growth opportunities I had with his company. He is a gentleman of the highest integrity and honour and it was my privilege to have served him for over two decades. That is the story of how I went from the company's top performer, to out the door on a retrenchment tide not six months later. I did remain for a full month after the other unsuccessful applicants had departed. I had been asked to create a Wikipedia-style intranet document detailing what I did, how I did it and anything else my successor would need to know. I still don't know how to say no.

Life Lessons:

- It's time to start prioritising me
- Nothing lasts forever
- If you want loyalty, get a dog

Chapter 27

The what now conundrum

For a couple of weeks, I celebrated my freedom. I slept until I was ready to get up, went out for coffee with girlfriends, I joined the other ladies that lunch and I was good, still missing half my vocabulary and in terrible pain, but good. Then one morning I woke up and I couldn't get out of bed.

I had no strength at all. I slid onto the floor and crawled to the bathroom. When I turned on the shower, the water felt like hot needles piercing my skin. I battled to draw breath and every inhalation hurt. My eyes burned and watered, my body ached, my legs felt heavy, I trembled, my ears rang and buzzed and I felt as though someone had poured lead into me. I dragged myself back onto my bed and lay there in my wet towel all day, because I didn't have the energy to get dressed. I stayed in that state for almost an entire year.

A successful day was one where I could shower, dress and feed the dogs. If I dropped something on the floor, it stayed there until someone came to visit me. If I bent down, I fell over, so I didn't bend. It was always nice to see people, but the added strain of trying to hide my frailty was unbearable. The only way my brain was clear enough to think and form words, was if I was lying down. I saw fewer and fewer people as the months rolled by until I was living like a hermit.

My old school friend who had sent me my beloved horse, was suffering from a Rickettsia infection and she was insistent that I had the same thing. Our symptoms mirrored and she wanted me to go onto something called the Jardin protocol. This is a protocol involving pulse antibiotic therapy with a combination of three different antibiotics at a time, taken for ten days each month. Different combinations of antibiotics would be used each month and treatment went on sometimes for years before patient's symptoms abated.

Treatment set up a massive Herxheimer reaction in most patients that amplified and, in some cases, added to their symptoms. This was from the toxins emitted by the dead bacteria. This might explain the old adage sometimes you have to get worse, before you can get better. Not all patients recover, but there have been some marvellously encouraging success stories using this protocol. Treatment is often combined with supportive vitamin and mineral therapies, dietary changes, saunas and so many other things. My friend was doing really well on the treatment and encouraged me to follow the regime.

Rickettsia infections are caused by exposure to tick borne bacteria. There are many different bacteria from many different ticks. As children we had ridden our horses and spent long hours on the farm. We were always pulling ticks off ourselves and the horses. We also swam the horses in filthy dam water and it turned out that our favourite place to go and lie in the grass and stare up at the sky, was an old tick research foundation premises. It all seemed to fit.

The only problem with this diagnosis was that lab tests for tick born infections are notorious for giving false negatives, which mine naturally were and no one really believed these chronic conditions actually existed in South Africa. I have spoken to so many doctors about Rickettsia and Lyme disease and without exception they have said, "We don't get those in this country." One doctor told me that all he had been taught about Rickettsia at university was covered in one short paragraph. If you were diagnosed with tick bite fever you were given antibiotics for a week and that was that.

My friend had done so much research and had uncovered some horrific stories about weaponised tick bacteria from the second world war, hush campaigns from leading health organisations and a whole mess of crap. I'm not going into this here because that is another fight, for another day, by another crusader. How this relates to my story, however, is that this turned out to be yet another blind alley. Another life-limiting diagnosis that I accepted on anecdotal evidence alone, out of sheer desperation to have a name for the demons that plagued me. I could not follow the protocol she was on, because the doctor who ran it was in a different part of the country and I couldn't get to her.

Also, the tests were prohibitively expensive and I no longer had an income. I spent months lying in bed, reading articles and researching Rickettsia and its American cousin Lyme disease on my iPad. I was convinced this was the answer I had been looking for my whole life. Rickettsia infection comes with a host of co-infections. I eventually, years later, tested positive for past exposure to many of the co-infections such as mycoplasma pneumonia, chlamydia pneumonia and so on, but I tested negative for the actual Rickettsia bacteria. During my year long stint in bed however, I was convinced I had the answer. I learned that chronic infections from these agents causes the body to be depleted of vitamins and minerals and a general collapse of the immune system was responsible for almost all of my symptoms. I had been told by more than one alternative practitioner using bio-feedback mechanisms that I was vitamin and mineral deplete, one went so far as to say, "You may be grossly overweight, but you are starving to death." Nice!

I eventually found a doctor who called himself an integrative physician. He acknowledged the existence of Rickettsia and he had a Quantum Scio machine that actually picked up the Rickettsia when I was tested. SCIO stands for Scientific Consciousness Interface Operating System. This is a biofeedback device that detects stressors in the body, then emits healthy patterns back to the body, balancing it at the subtle energy level. The SCIO was developed by William C Nelson during the 1970's. This doctor, however, didn't believe in using antibiotics unless absolutely necessary and he was certainly not going to prescribe them three at a time for years on end.

He adjusted my diet and loaded me up with supplements to try and correct all the depletions. He used something called a Rife machine which is also a part of the frequency-based medicine this doctor practised alongside his regular medical skills. Dr Raymond Rife invented his machine during the 1920-1930's. He identified the electrical frequency of a multitude of pathogens, bacteria, viruses, fungi and parasites and worked out what frequency would destroy them.

To make sense of this weird shit, think of an opera singer who can sing a note so high, that it can shatter glass and you have the right image for Rife. I was sceptical, but after I had consulted the doctor about a septic ingrown toenail problem, I became a believer. After my big holiday Humpty Dumpty impersonation, one of my broken toes had healed slightly twisted and crooked and the nail was constantly ingrown and painful. I had ignored this as I did with most things as far as possible, until one day I noticed my entire big toe had turned black. I dragged myself to the doctor and he agreed that, for this, he would prescribe an antibiotic, but first I was to try the Rife machine. Well colour me stunned when the next morning I woke up to a pink, happy looking toe!

So, there I was, diagnosed once again, with an unconfirmed, (except for a bio-feedback machine that isn't recognised by the medical fraternity at large) life-limiting condition. I spent a fortune on supplements and homeopathic solutions, naturopathic treatments and I even went so far as to buy a Rife machine and a home-use bio-feedback device. Did I feel any better? I went from operating at around ten percent capacity, to around twenty percent capacity. A vast improvement relative to my state of incapacity, that gave me some hope. However, it went so far and no further and I remained largely bed ridden, and unable to work.

Life Lessons:

- When you really crash, it's nearly impossible to get up again
- Getting up, dressing up and showing up are all actually optional
- Having a medical degree doesn't guarantee knowledge
- Alternative therapies help, but only to a point
- Frequency medicine is interesting

Chapter 28

The enough is enough conundrum

I'm starting to lose faith in the whole Rickettsia idea. My friend was adamant that I needed to do her treatment, but I didn't have access to it. I'm actually very grateful for that, since years later when I finally managed to get myself tested, I tested negative for Rickettsia. I was so desperate at the time I would have taken those massive amounts of drugs even without testing. What I was doing with the integrative physician, whilst clearly supporting my body in some ways, was not giving me back my life. I had been over six months on treatment and the improvement wasn't enough to instil confidence. I still spent most of my days in bed, or resting, I was still in pain and my brain was mush.

My integrative doctor, whilst being a lovely man, kept giving me multi-vitamins, milk thistle, omega three, vitamin D and at each visit a let's try this component or two to try for the next month. He remained non-committal, and I was getting frustrated and feeling ignored again. I called for an appointment one day, when something out of the ordinary had me feeling worse than usual. His receptionist told me he was on leave. I asked her who looked after his patients in that scenario (most doctors have a locum, or they buddy up with a colleague at a different practice). She snapped at me, "Doctor is entitled to take leave, you will just have to get on with it and wait until he returns." Well he may have returned, but I didn't.

I read an article on dealing with loss of function. How to cope in a wheelchair. Dear God! I didn't want to end up in a wheelchair, but I confess, I was afraid I might not ever recover. Perhaps that was what my future looked like. The article advised me to stop focussing on my recovery and to write up a list of Big Sexy End Goals. A statement of intent as it were. Things that I really wanted and things I could do from within the confines of my condition (whatever that might be).

Here's my list:

- My body is pain free (well that's a no brainer)

- I would like to be a motivational speaker – I love public speaking, and I believe in the power of people – perhaps not myself, but other people certainly.
- I want to deliver a TED Talk – (I was a member of Toastmasters Int for a while and I can deliver a mean talk.
- I want to teach workshops – I've always loved the teaching aspects of anything I've done – I love sharing and empowering people.
- I want financial abundance – well who doesn't – plus I'm unemployed, and currently unemployable.
- I want to travel overseas – well, of course I do, it's the ultimate reward. Ireland and Italy for sure. Mauritius any day of the week.
- I want to write best-selling books that help people – I've needed so much help in life – there are probably others out there just like me.
- I want to write a children's book – I love children, and reading to my girls was always such a special time – there's something magical about a child with a book.
- I want to weigh 74kg in good health – When I fell pregnant with my first child, I weighed 78kg. I was 88kg when I went into labour, and 74kg when I came home from the hospital – I always loved being 74kg.
- I want to be a fun, loving grandmother – grand kids!! – Yes please, lots of them. Let's have a noisy, happy family home again.
- I want to support my children's lives in a meaningful way – they are grown women and I no longer have the right to tell them what to do, or how to live their lives. My opinions are simply that, my opinions. I always want to be there for them however, in whatever capacity I can, and I will wait to find out what is meaningful for them.
- I want to allow myself to be loved and adored – I've never felt safe enough to be vulnerable enough to accept love. I have some serious trust issues.

When I read that list now, it makes me part sad and part proud. What I did realise though, was that all of that could be achieved whether I could walk or not. I was starting to build the possibility of a new future that could be tailored to my needs and not based on anyone else's needs or expectations. Also, by realising that life wouldn't stop if I remained incapacitated, I began to lose the fear of incapacitation, thus releasing myself to begin to recover.

I was reading everything I could find and was researching ways to help with the chronic fatigue and the fibromyalgia at least, if not the Rickettsia. Oddly enough the crossover of symptoms with the three diagnoses is startling. I read up on balanced health methods and realised I needed to get myself moving again. I made an appointment at the local gym for an assessment with a bio kineticist. Who better to help me regain my strength and flexibility, than an exercise specialist? I also decided to sign up with a therapist to address the mental aspects of my health. I still did not feel depressed, but I was most definitely miserable. I felt so alone in this mess and I'd had enough of lying around waiting to see whether I would live or die; waiting and hoping that someone else might save me. I needed an action plan and I needed to take control. My inner warrior who had been AWOL for a long time got up, dressed up and showed up. About bloody time too.

I started my rehabilitation by walking with my Great Dane. He had lain next to me for months with his head resting on my belly, gazing at me lovingly. He would go outside to piddle and then climb right back onto my bed and stay with me. He was the most dependable thing in my life. He would lie with his head on my shoulder some days and I could feel the love emanating from him and washing over me. I told him we had a mission to get me walking again and he wagged his tail encouraging me. He was a very old boy himself by then at nine years of age. The average life span for a Great Dane is seven. His brother had sadly passed away already and I knew he wasn't long for this life.

I put on his lead and we tottered out of the front gate. I took five or six steps across the road. Feeling dizzy, I panicked and we went back to bed. Each day we managed a few more steps. He walked beside me quietly and never once pulled or tugged on his lead. I felt safe with him. He waited patiently, while I puffed and panted at the corner, trying to decide whether I could go on or needed to go back. He calmly accepted my decision. Within two weeks we are walking around the block. I am still not confident enough to add the sausage dog into the mix, because he barks maniacally and pulls like a mini steam train.

Being more mobile, I could now set up some sessions with the therapist. She lived down the road from me. Easy to get to, easy access to her rooms, no long walks needed, parking right outside the door. I didn't have much energy and I guarded it carefully and expended it judiciously. I wasn't sure if I liked her or not, she spent a lot of time telling me about her past relationship drama that had caused her to lose weight and I wasn't sure how that was relevant to me. But she had a

Rife machine and put me onto the depression programme. Exactly which pathogen causes depression I do not know, but okay I would see how things progressed. I still had days where I could not get out of bed. I seemed to take one step forward, two sideways, and one backwards. But I made it a point everyday, to get up and get dressed, no matter if I lay on the couch all day, that became my new baseline.

I'd had a few bad days and I was keen to get outside again, so clutching my dog's lead, I headed off for a big field about three blocks away. If I could get there, I could let my boy have a free run and a good sniff while I sat under a tree. We made it and I got a bit cocky. I left the safety of the perimeter fence and followed the track around. Suddenly my legs gave way under me and I crumpled to the ground. My dog ran over and immediately lay down next to me with his head on my shoulder. I was a bit stunned. I took my time gathering my wits and when I tried to get up, I had no strength in me. My arms were too weak to push myself up and my legs just wouldn't cooperate.

It took me about fifteen minutes to wobble myself upright. I headed cautiously for the fence and was halfway there, when I fell again. This time it took even longer to get up. My dog stayed right beside me all the way. By now the tears were pouring down my face. I was shaking like a leaf and I have never felt so wretched. But it didn't end there. We eventually left the field and I was shuffling along at a rate of one centimetre per step, when my legs gave out for a third time. I lay on the pavement in the baking sun for almost an hour. Four cars drove past me and a couple of pedestrians walked past on the opposite side of the road.

I sure had this invisibility lark down pat. I know people sometimes get so self-absorbed they don't see what's going on around them and everyone is running around with extremely busy and important lives, but here I was a large, overweight woman lying face down on the pavement, sobbing, with a giant black dog lying next to me… and no one saw me? No one stopped. No one offered to help me. I felt like I was the only person on the planet who even knew I was alive and I wondered what I was even living for.

I couldn't dance, I couldn't sing, I couldn't ride, my children were grown and had left home, I couldn't work and now it seemed I couldn't even walk. My future seemed so bleak and I once again began to wonder if it was time to end it all. A bead of sweat ran down my face and into the corner of my eye and it burned like a bitch! I jabbed at it with my dirty fingers, covered in sand from scabbling in the dirt to get up and it hurt even more. Now both of my eyes were on fire. It wasn't enough that I was prostrate on the street, the Universe seemed to delight in toying with me and there seemed to be no end to the layers of torment levied in my direction. Mother must have been right all along; I must be a really terrible person to be attracting this level of shit!

I took a juddering breath, lip trembling, the picture of abject misery and suddenly something went click inside my brain and I got mad. I became incensed. I swore out loud at every God I could think of, "Enough already, you bloody great bully. Leave me the fuck alone!!!! You think I'm going to lie here and die in the dirt like an abandoned dog, well you can bloody well think again!!!" And with that I heaved myself unsteadily to my feet and my beautiful dog led me, shuffling slowly, safely home.

I had an appointment with the therapist the next day which I was very pleased about. I felt as though I had reached a crisis point and I wanted to talk it through with someone objective. I started to tell her my story about how I had fallen in the field the first time. She interrupted me and said, "Well clearly you are a very clumsy person…". I didn't stay for the end of the sentence. I shuffled out of there at high speed, fuelled by a rage and indignation that powered my recalcitrant legs. We were done! She had the temerity to send me a bill for the session and my inner ten-month-old made another live appearance and said, "Well fuck you too!" Is there no one who will give me the time of day, not even for payment. Well, sorry for you lady, no time, no pay! Wherever I go, it would seem I am at fault. People just do not see me… even when I am screaming from the rooftops and waving my arms, trying desperately to show myself to them.

The next stop was the gym. The bio kineticist was late for my appointment and I sat in the waiting area in that noisy, high energy gymnasium to wait for him. My nervous system twitched from the over stimulation of the lights, the music and the multitudes of people. Eventually after fifteen minutes my name was called by a young man standing miles away from me on a staircase. He called out to me to, "Hurry up, I don't have all day to wait for you."

All heads swivelled in my direction and people gawked at me as I struggled to get to my feet. The receptionist had told me to sit in the wrong place to wait for him and he had been looking for me and was clearly annoyed. Well I was pretty damned annoyed too. Here I was, easily four times the size of every other patron, dressed in baggy clothes, while they were all sleek in their designer gym gear, hair slicked back with sweat from their strenuous workouts, sipping power smoothies and sporting sweat towels and gym bags, and now I had to try and climb up the stairs to the second floor for my assessment, with them all staring at me. I clutched onto the railings and slowly hauled myself up, one painful stair at a time. My legs were so swollen that my knees couldn't bend properly. Sweat was pouring down my face and back. By the time I got to the top I was shaking like a leaf. This arrogant young man had a really bad attitude when he asked me why I was there. Wasn't it obvious?

Calming myself and quelling the desire to wring his stupid little neck; he was less than half my age and was talking to me like I was an annoying child; I explained that I had been ill and had been bed ridden for an extended period and I was interested in being rehabilitated. I wanted to regain my strength and balance and needed some help with that. This seemed to irritate him even more and he let out a deep sigh and said, "Alright get down on the floor and do some sit ups, let's see what you can do." Had he not heard a word I'd said? I could no more get down on the floor and do a bloody sit up than I could fly to the moon.

If I could get down on the floor and up again, unaided, I wouldn't need anyone to help me. If I could do a sit up, I could probably conquer the world. "I can't get down without something to hold onto," I ventured. "This session is over!" he snapped. "You can't even arrive on time and now you won't even try. I can't waste my time on you. I suggest you go home and get back into bed. There's nothing to be done for you." Well I had two choices, shrivel up and die right there, or find my own way out of the darkness. I did a quick mental check in with my inner ten-month-old and, delighted to be given airtime, she said... that's right, you've guessed it, "Well fuck you too!!!!!!!!!"

I signed up for an exorbitantly expensive gym contract, donned a swimming costume and lowered my weak, flabby, oversized bulk into the kiddies' pool; where the elderly ladies did their aquacise classes. In the beginning all I did was walk up and down in the water. Within two months however, I was in the big pool swimming twenty-five metre lengths. Within three months I was swimming forty lengths a day. My biggest nemesis remained the aluminium ladder getting in and out of the pool. I was wider than it allowed for and the sharp steps hurt my painful feet. Then the money ran out and I had to relinquish my gym membership in favour of paying for things like electricity and dog food.

Life Lessons:

- No matter how bad it gets, with the right attitude you can always find your way back
- Baby steps are to be celebrated

Weird Shit!

- It is possible to live life at a measured pace and not at a hundred miles an hour
- There is an entire world in the space between all and nothing
- I'm in this on my own
- My dog is my biggest support
- It's better to fight for yourself, than to waste time fighting against injustice and ignorance

Chapter 29

The can you really go back conundrum

Whilst I had been lying in my bed, I had received a friend request on social media from my old Wholism Healing teacher. I was delighted to hear from her and we started meeting for coffee dates. At this stage, since we were no longer teacher and student, we began to form a friendship. I loved hearing her stories about the energy work she was doing and I found it still thrilled me to my core. She remained in awe of the work I had done at the rehab centre and that part of me that had been shamed into silence began to stir again.

I think this woman was the only one in my whole life at that point, who looked at me and didn't flinch from what she saw. She didn't see someone who was a problem to be fixed, clumsy and overweight, or bitter and frustrated, washed up and useless; she saw me, warts and all and she treated me as though I was perfectly normal. I didn't need to pretend to be anyone else with her. With all my flaws and limitations, I was still a powerful, interesting, valid woman in her eyes. It didn't matter to her that I couldn't hold down a nine to five job; that on a good day I had perhaps four functional hours available to me and then I needed to rest; that I was a shadow of my former self; that my brain was a traitorous swine that hid words from me and turned me into a linguistic buffoon; that I had no functional purpose in the real world. She saw what was right with me, what value I did have, and I determined to start seeing myself that way too.

I took a little part time job in a factory shop. It was menial work and it was horrendous. I had been tasked with suggesting improvements and many were needed. The premises were filthy, the office staff were horrid. The other part timer was pleasant enough, but if I tidied up and moved things around to make them more efficient, she moved everything back. I had been asked to make improvements, but everything I did was simply reversed. If I offered a suggestion, I was told that wasn't the way they did things. I couldn't wait to get out of there. They say you can do anything if you are desperate enough, well I would like to heartily disagree with that. I could no more sit in that grubby little cubicle answering customers dumb questions all day, for minimum wage, than I could govern a country.

I was berated on a daily basis by customers who had not been able to find parking. Screamed at when the credit card machine went down, held accountable for the hot temperature in the little shop; and my goodness, let something not be available after they had parked a mile away, then I would never hear the end of it. The point of sale machine was so old and buggered that I would ring up a string of goodies and realise that half of them hadn't been input. I went too quickly for the machine. The printing pad on the till slips was problematic and the slips often came out blank or so faint one couldn't read them. It was a nightmare. I found point of sale companies and suggested them to the office ladies, who told me to do my job and mind my own business.

A customer asked me one day, "I'm doing fillet steak for a dinner party tonight. Do you think my guests would prefer pepper sauce or mushroom sauce?" Well, my inner voice is heavily sarcastic and anyone who knows anything about food knows that the right answer to that question is tomato sauce (ketchup) so… Or my other favourite, "Do you think this spice will be spicy enough for my husband?" How the hell should I know? "When will the bulk cake mixes be available?" Well, since there was no production schedule available for me to look up and no one in the factory appeared to have that information, if indeed I could find anyone to answer the phone in the first place, I sat there looking like an idiot, representing this company and brand and not being able to answer customers questions or find out the answers for them. Not a good representation at all. For someone who prides herself on being extremely proactive and was used to managing a large online shopping mall, it was beyond frustrating. At the end of my short-term contract I lit out of there like my bum was on fire and I never looked back.

One or two customers however, I did connect with. Thank goodness, or perhaps it was by cosmic design, the shop was deserted at the time. One lady came and stood at the till point and she seemed perfectly normal. She was well dressed, she smiled when she spoke, but she had the saddest eyes I had ever seen. I stopped ringing up her purchases and said to her, "You are so brave the way you are carrying on with life. Please remember though to take time out to feel how you truly feel."

Sometimes I wonder who puts the words in my mouth. She looked at me with wide eyes and as her tears spilled down her cheeks, she deflated and fell into a chair. She put her head down on the counter and she sobbed. No one came into the normally busy shop, the phone didn't ring, no one disturbed us. She sobbed for about ten minutes and then looked up with a ravaged expression and told me her story.

Her son had been diagnosed with end stage cancer. He lived overseas and he had wanted to protect her from any distress his condition might cause her so he never told her he was ill. He had finally called though to ask her to come to him. He was at the end of his road. He was scared and he needed his mom. In a state of shock, she had hopped onto the first available flight. She didn't make it in time and he passed away before she got to him.

Her life had disintegrated in one day and she had no way of connecting to the horror of what had happened. She hadn't had time to process the idea of her child being ill, let along losing her precious boy. She hadn't had time to tell him how much she loved him and how being his mom had been the highlight of her life. She never got to say goodbye. That had been three months prior, and that day, in that grubby little shop, was the first time she had cried for him.

Another lady came in and she had a personality a mile wide. I grinned just looking at her. She had an infectious laugh and she was quite the jolliest person I had ever met. For some reason I felt compelled to tell her that my sister in law had had a stroke. Again, I wonder who puts the words in my mouth. Well every ounce of jolly evaporated and she became quite the angriest woman I had seen in a long while. She was really up close and personal in that tiny little shop, which thank goodness, once again remained quiet and deserted.

She ranted and raved and vented her spleen and she had a lot to be angry about. She had married early in life and her husband had died suddenly of a heart attack only one year into their marriage. Her second husband had had a stroke and he too passed away soon after marrying. Her third husband, it turned out was a big mistake. Whereas she had loved the first two passionately, she married the third one for companionship. It transpired that after the first flush of excitement had passed, she really didn't like him very much at all. She was making plans to leave him when he too suffered a massive stroke.

He was alive, locked in silence, unable to do anything for himself and she was mad. She hadn't signed on to be a nurse, she wanted to live and to travel. She had a business over in Ireland that was going to ruin because she couldn't get there. She was so frustrated and her emotions reminded me of the whirling dervishes I had seen in Dubai. She felt too guilty to leave him. She felt too angry and cheated by life to look after him, and she was well and truly stuck.

She had gone to play bowls one day and had taken hubby along in his wheelchair. He was struck by lightning! The karma this woman was working with must have been huge. He didn't die though, oh no, he actually regained his power of speech. You would think that this inexplicable medical miracle would have been cause for celebration, but sadly it was not so. She had taken full advantage of the fact that he couldn't talk back and she had made her feelings about looking after him perfectly clear. If this little vent session was anything to go by, she certainly didn't mince her words and the poor bugger must have received a serious earful over the years. They say payback is a bitch and I think this lady would agree.

One thing I did realise from the many customer interactions, where it seemed I was acting as some sort of catalyst for their repressed emotions; I was meant to get back into the energy work. I went back to Wholism Healing, which had been rebranded as Inner Tuition. I agreed to co-facilitate a course with my friend. I dived back in and I never looked back. I loved this work, but I still wasn't able to start practising, because I couldn't stand for the full hour while I did a session with a client. I had about five minutes of standing in my unreliable legs.

I was managing to create the illusion of having a life, but I was always mindful of my need to sit. If there were no chairs, I couldn't be there. If there was walking involved, I couldn't go. I worked out which shops had parking right outside, were all on one level, had trolleys for me to lean on and had small, easily remembered floor plans. I could scoot in and do a fast shop and get out again before my legs gave out. I knew what time of day the queues were shortest and I shopped then and only then.

I had to give away concert tickets because I knew I couldn't walk from the car to the stadium and I wouldn't manage the stairs once inside. Also, I would not be able to sit on a hard seat for hours on end. That was a bit of a low point for me. There were many invitations I had to decline and understandably so, I received less and less invitations to spend time with old friends. But in spite of that, I was having a wonderful time working with the new students and sharing my experiences. It made me laugh when they all looked stunned and amazed as the story of Inner Tuition was explained to them. I watched them make connections not previously considered and thrilled in sharing with them how vast and magical the world of energy really is.

When we began to apply what we were teaching practically and they felt the energy for themselves, their responses were always amusing. Some really weird shit went down every single time. I have never met a student who did not gain a world of insight from doing those courses. Not all of them wanted to work with energy. For many it was a stand alone experience. It didn't matter though as seeds were planted and receptors for understanding were triggered. At some stage in their lives, when the time was right for them, they would be able to draw from what they had learned. For the most part though, these students became wiser, stronger, more authentic versions of themselves.

Without even a menial job to bolster my finances, the funds soon ran dry. I was in a bit of a state about it. I was spending a fortune on supplements, herbal remedies, medical tests, doctors, alternative practitioners… anything I could think of to try and find my way back to full health. I didn't really see how I could continue to keep my home afloat. Then the unimaginable happened. My beautiful Great Dane looked me in the eye one day and he let me know, in no uncertain terms, that his work here was done and he needed to leave this earthly plane.

I was back on my feet again, albeit in a diminished capacity and it was time for him to rest. With the heaviest of hearts my family gathered and we took him to the beach for one last hurrah. He stood with the sun on his face, his giant soft velvety ears flapping in the breeze, gazing across the ocean at the mountains in the distance and I knew that he was already there in Spirit, running free. I hugged him and told him that he was the love of my life. I thanked him for being the most incredible companion anyone could ever wish for. The vet came to the house the next day. Snuggled on his favourite couch, wrapped in my favourite blanket, he was allowed to go to his final rest.

I was bereft. After a paralysing period of grieving, I had to face the facts. I could no longer afford to live in my home. I spoke to ex-Husband about it one day when he popped in for a visit. Either I had to take in boarders, or I had to leave the country and go to the UK and live on benefits. I couldn't work as I couldn't be sure from one day to the next whether I could even get out of bed, let alone leave the house. I was still only operating at around forty percent capacity.

My retirement planning had been cut short by fifteen years and so wouldn't amount to a hill of beans, I had lost all the group life cover I had when I left the office, which still annoys me no end. I had moved my provident fund across, but it wasn't enough to live on. We discussed me moving into his spare room and renting out my house. Well that solved the financial issues, but it raised a few new ones. Can you ever really go back? All the reasons we had divorced were still valid and in play, but I didn't see that I had a choice. However, housemate is a very different dynamic to marriage partner, so, figuring any port in a storm, with a grateful heart, I moved in (after I had gutted and renovated the place of course, because... well because it just needed to be done!)

Life Lessons:

- A teacher can become a friend and a colleague
- In the world of weird shit, I have value
- You can't do just anything in life, not if you want to stay sane
- Everyone is hiding something behind their mask
- There's always a way back
- People and animals come into your life for a reason, a season, or a need
- You can go back, just on different terms

Chapter 30

The stress conundrum

I was feeling pretty good about myself. My financial worries were now manageable. I was physically safe and secure. I had reached a place of acceptance with my health and I had paused in my desperate search for answers. I was working on being grateful for the functionality I did have and I was trying to live the best life I could with what I had. I still carried huge amounts of grief for the life I had lost and all that was no longer available to me, but my focus was firmly forward. I had the odd relapse where I would try a new doctor or pursue a new theory, but for the most part I kept my eyes forward and tried to be grateful for what I had.

If things got too claustrophobic living with ex-Husband, I could go out of town and visit with my sister; or go to my old school bestie who lived in the bush. I had been so enamoured of her lifestyle the first time I went to stay, that I couldn't wait to get back. The bush veld was a completely different world to the one I inhabited and I loved it. It was so much more rugged and real. The people were more friendly and less judgemental than town folk, although they did thrive on gossip. They laughed good naturedly at my pathetic attempts to speak Afrikaans and always spoke to me in English which I really appreciated.

One day whilst visiting in the bush, I found myself involved in a darting and relocation exercise of the wild game. My friend farms Livingstone eland as well as cattle. Some of the eland were being relocated to a different farm and others needed vaccinations and genetic testing. Game capture is a very testosterone driven, high stakes process, with khaki clad rugged men, who drive big white off-road vehicles, all shouting at one another.

Once an animal is darted, everyone becomes laser focused to ensure nothing untoward happens to it. These valuable animals are processed and woken up again with the minimum of interference and in the shortest possible time. The air is fraught with tension until the last precious animal has been woken up, or safely loaded onto the game truck. My job was to take photographs and to record the measurements of the horns, the vaccination numbers and so on. It was thrilling. My friend was hugely amused at how excited I was. What to me, was an incredible adventure, to her, was just life.

Another area of her life that fascinated me was her warthogs. She had been given an abandoned baby warthog to raise. Typically, as with any rescue situation one became two, two became three... I think to date she has rescued around ten or so of these amazing animals. Five of them live on her property and while they were growing up and needed bottle feeding, they lived in the house. The first one, Twiggy was about a year and a half old when I met her. The second one, Charlie, was around three months old. Twiggy took one look at me and declared war. She shoved me on my arm with her rock-hard snout and my bones jarred. She earned my instant respect and complete wariness.

For some reason she hated me on sight, and she delighted in sneaking up behind me and squealing. I swear she laughed out loud as I ran for my life. I unleashed my inner athlete on more than one occasion, seeking refuge from the enraged hog by clambering up onto the table or diving over the back of the couch. She never ever did a thing to me in front of my friend, but she was a worthy adversary. I'll swear she was a closet assassin. I was utterly enchanted, scared witless, but enchanted.

The experience was just so rich and I couldn't keep it to myself. With my friend's kind permission, I settled down to write my children's book. I called it Warthog Tales and was delighted to have it published. My friend is also a prolific writer of short stories and musings that she shares on social media, much to the delight of her hundreds of followers. I find her life to be truly fascinating and really felt that her story should be shared. She dominates in a traditionally masculine world without losing one ounce of her femininity. She is proof positive that you can achieve anything if you set your mind to it and don't take no for an answer. I offered to collate and edit her stories into a book for her. After trawling through three or four years of Facebook posts to collect the stories and editing the articles to remove emoji speak, we had such fun compiling this manuscript. She too received a publication offer, although she has yet to publish.

One day while I was writing, my daughter called me from Cape Town. She was driving to an appointment. While we were chatting on the phone, she was car jacked. All I heard was her window being smashed and her screaming, then a rhythmic sound. On calm reflection it was probably the phone's speaker rubbing on a jacket pocket as the thief ran off, but to my terrified mind it was the sound of my beloved child being raped and murdered.

I must interject here that a student at the school where my other daughter teaches had been attacked by thugs, intent on stealing her mobile phone. She was jogging in the forest just a short distance from her mother and sister when she was attacked. They stole her phone after raping and murdering her. My daughters and I had joined our community and walked a silent vigil through the forest in solidarity with the girl's parents and sibling. It remains to this day one of the most difficult things I have ever done. No one wants to be that close to such intimate grief. This trauma was still fairly fresh in my mind and when I heard my child scream, I went to the darkest of places.

My daughter, thank goodness, was unharmed. She had managed to drive away with the thug half inside her car and apart from losing her phone and her bag, having her car window smashed and being very shaken up, she was relatively unscathed. Hysterical with fear, I ran straight through a closed security gate and tore it right off the hinges to get to my friend. The poor woman had no idea how to reach me, such was the enormity of my shock and horror. I had gone to a place so dark and terrifying I didn't think I would ever get back. She took the phone from me, listened and said, "I can't hear her, she isn't there anymore." All I heard was she is gone, she is dead.

I contacted my friend from Inner Tuition who had a small band of energy workers who offered their services for emergency healing and she put out a request for them to help me. She described my energy field as being shattered beyond recognition, almost as though it was confetti that had been blown about by a strong wind. It took considerable effort to rebuild my energy field and I was left in a state that could be equated to being held together with tape and glue.

In the days and weeks after this terrifying incident, I began to fall apart. I lay in my room at the opposite end of the house to my friend and night after night I suffered with rolling panic attacks. My heart raced, I sweated and shook uncontrollably, I had chest pains and I felt dizzy. I became terrified of everything. I imagined snakes were writhing across my floor, bugs were coming in every crack and crevice and I was a wreck.

Unfortunately, in South Africa we have a very unstable political situation. Farm attacks are at an all-time high as repatriation of land is promised by the politicians. Terror attacks are a nightly occurrence. Every morning my friend would fill me in on the details of the latest farm attack and resultant murders that had happened overnight; all of which were occurring within a two-hour driving radius of where we were staying. It all became too much.

Then I developed an ear infection that morphed into cellulitis. When my face and scalp swelled hot and angry and the doctor wanted to hospitalise me for ten days intravenous antibiotic treatment, I threw in the towel and flew back home. What followed was just diabolical. I went to see a physician and explained my symptoms to him. He ran an ECG and ordered dozens of blood and urine tests and he sent me for an MRI scan. His treadmill stopped working during the ECG and he couldn't get the report to print out, but he said he was satisfied that he hadn't seen anything while I had been puffing along, so he was happy to call it fine and move on.

The MRI report said raised intercranial pressure. The physician sent me to a neurosurgeon, who gave me possibly, the most comprehensive medical consultation I had ever had. He said he could see four white flares on the scan. If there were six or more, he would say I had multiple sclerosis, but because there were only four it didn't mean anything. Well I don't know how many people would be happy with that assumption, I know I wasn't. He admitted that he wasn't the right guy to read the scan, he simply operated on whatever was diagnosed. He wondered why I had come to see him. Well... because I was sent by the physician!

He suggested I see a neurologist for final diagnosis. I did just that and the neurologist told me I had the brain of a young girl. I asked him why I had such trouble remembering words and why I struggled so with my memory. I had by this stage lost large chunks of my life story, I simply could not remember. He said it was because I was a bored, overweight housewife. He saw women like me all the time. I should get a hobby to stimulate me. My memories were all still there and I would remember when I was sufficiently motivated to do so. "Well fuck you too!"

I went back to see the physician, still suffering with every symptom. He started the consultation by asking me if I was taking the medication I had been prescribed. I told him I was. He asked me about a tablet I wasn't on. When I told him that, he got quite agitated and said he knew he had given it me because it was written down in my folder. I leaned over and looked at the folder in front of him. It belonged to a male patient and it was nothing to do with me.

He then called in his receptionist and shouted at her in front of me for her sloppy filing; and for making him look bad (in my opinion he was doing a good job of that all on his own). After that really uncomfortable incident, he took a phone call and arranged dinner plans with his wife. He shuffled papers on his desk and looked at my proper file (the poor harangued receptionist had delivered it in the interim) and then he started to complain because I'd had so many tests done.

He launched into a long lecture about my weight. I told him that I had battled for years to shift the weight and gave him a little of my history. He said, "The only solution for someone like you, is to have a gastric band fitted, but since you are too weak to withstand the surgery, there isn't anything that can be done for you." He then went on to say that he didn't have the time or the inclination to write up a report for my GP because of the large number of tests I'd had (which he had ordered); and since there wasn't anything wrong with me anyway, I should just carry on and see him in a month.

Okay, so on one hand, I was too weak to withstand a lifesaving surgery, but on the other hand there was nothing wrong with me. Well I don't know anyone who has back to back panic attacks all night long, is permanently drenched in sweat and who shakes uncontrollably, all in perfect health, but alrighty then. Since there was nothing wrong with me, why on earth should I make another appointment? I didn't.

Any port in a storm being my default back up plan, I went to see the hairy therapist. Thinking I was going mad, I decided to consult someone in the know. He listened to my story and said, "You have classic PTSD." Post-traumatic stress disorder was something I associated with war veterans. He assured me it was a much more common problem than that and I indeed was suffering from it. He proceeded to hypnotise me and the glorious result of that one session, was that all of my symptoms stopped. It was as though he had reached inside of me and switched something off. I was no longer in a state of ongoing panic, I could breathe again. While I still had a mild tremor, the uncontrollable shaking had stopped. After three and a half months of exhausting, debilitating, symptoms, it was nothing short of a miracle.

My sister invited me to come and stay with her to recuperate. She lived with her partner on a fishing lodge about forty kilometres outside of town. Her partner had been trying to get me to come and stay for a month. I had been for a couple of shorter visits, but he was adamant I should come for a month. It became a bit of a joke between us. On this occasion I was very happy to accept their offer. Their place was idyllic. No neighbours to be seen, no traffic, no noise. Their garden was the riverbank and there was nothing but peace and solitude for miles around. He would go fishing all day, then come home and cook the delicious freshly caught fish for our supper. I had my own private flat on the property and I slept solidly for almost two weeks. One day I woke up and I just knew I was better.

We had a wonderful day together and that evening we toasted my recovery. In the middle of the night, my sister came banging on my door. Her partner had gotten up to go to the bathroom and had collapsed. I hurried inside and found him lying naked on the floor with blood pooled around his head. He had struck his nose when he fell. He was making a terrible gurgling sound, but when I touched his body, I could feel that he was gone. I covered him with a blanket.

Telling my sister to get dressed and phone the nearest neighbour, who was a fishing buddy of her partner, I went back to my flat, where I calmly washed my hair and got dressed. I felt completely in control, but I needed to have my hair straight to face what was coming. Such comfort in the utter mundane. My poor sister was in a deep state of shock. The neighbour had alerted everyone who lived up and down the river and had then come running, toting a rifle. He thought we had fallen foul of a farm attack; our country is in a bad way.

Being sensitive to the fact that this was his friend, I explained what had happened. Some other neighbours started arriving, one of them was a nursing sister. She confirmed that he had indeed passed away and everyone stood stunned, staring at each other. I heard myself take charge and I started issuing instructions. Someone was despatched to call the paramedics, others were sent to the end of the dust road to wave the paramedics in. The location of this lodge was incredibly difficult to find and access to the larger farm area was through a remote-controlled gate. Someone else was despatched to open the gate. Someone was to sit with my sister, others were to make tea. No self-respecting crisis would be complete in an Englishman's life without a pot of tea. I took my sister's phone and called his family, his sister overseas, his children, whom I had never met and I gave them the worst news of their lives. Somehow, I managed to keep everything in motion.

The paramedics arrived and made the official pronouncement. We then had to repeat the entire process with the funeral home guys who came to collect the body. I asked them to put his body on the bed and we arranged him so that his wound was not visible. I cleaned up the blood off the floor and then left my sister sitting with her dead partner. Her life had just ended and I didn't know how to help her. I comforted his children who had rushed out to the river lodge; bereft young adults who sobbed in the arms of a woman they had never met. I encouraged them to sit with their father and say their goodbyes.

I sent an SOS text to my group of Inner Tuition energy healers hoping that one of them would pick it up. I felt better just knowing that they were holding the energy for us. My friend whose own husband had passed away only a couple of months prior said that she was having a wonderful dream, when her late husband burst onto the dream scene telling her to wake up and check her phone because I needed her. Grumbling at having her delicious dream disturbed she duly did as he asked and was shocked to read my message. She rallied the troops and did a phenomenal job of supporting me energetically throughout the ordeal.

Four hours later the hearse left and the neighbours went back to their beds in a state of shock and disbelief. My sister and I sat outside for the rest of the night, stunned and shaking our heads, unable to fully accept what had just happened. We watched as the sun rose slowly in the east and I remember feeling so surprised that the world was still turning, the tides were still ebbing and flowing, the fish were still jumping. Nothing had changed in the world and yet the whole world had changed for my sister.

She couldn't move. I brought her coffee and then I went in and changed her bed linen. I washed the blood-stained sheets and pillows and anything that didn't come clean, I bagged up and hid in my flat so she wouldn't have to deal with it. The neighbour came back in the morning, he needed to talk, he needed to process the events of the night. I remember how he looked at me like a little lost boy and he said, "Thank God you were here. I didn't know what to do. I froze. You were a pillar of strength. If I ever had to go to war, I would want to go with you."

I have never been exposed to such a raw and devastating grief as I witnessed in my sister. I felt as though I was gazing into her naked soul and I had no right to be in that intimate space. I did what I had been taught to do when studying Inner Tuition, I simply held the energy while she slowly tried to make sense of what had happened. The funeral arrangements were made and the memorial was a day that is best forgotten. So many people came to pay their respects, but my sister and I stood outside of it all. We didn't know or connect with any of these people and I could see, even though she didn't at the time, that she would need to leave this place. These were not her people.

I had also been taught, that when a person passes into Spirit, their energy stays present for three days, almost like an adjustment period. People have often said they could still feel their loved ones after they had gone and I choose to believe that this is an explanation for that. For three days after he passed, at 5.30 p.m. which was the time he would come back from the day's fishing, we would smell him. It was so powerful. We would be sitting out on the deck and suddenly we both startled, looked down at the jetty and then at one another and the tears would fall afresh as we caught the scent of his cologne. On the third day

I had gone to pour my sister a drink and when I came back outside, she was in pieces. She said she had smelt him as usual and her chair had started to shake as though someone was trying to tip it. Then he was gone and we never smelt him again. I ended up staying for a month.

Life Lessons:

- Always make the best out of a bad situation
- Gratitude is a good way to live your life
- People live vastly different lives
- Town mouse and country mouse is a real thing
- Some crimes are just so heinous they affect the way you perceive life
- When the chips are down, I can be strong and useful
- Empathy is a powerful trait
- When the heart stops, the world ends
- The weird shit always seems to end up being right

Chapter 31

The how much more can there be conundrum

I had a friend whom I had met at the office. I helped him work through his divorce trauma and we had become good buddies. He would change broken lights and drill holes if something needed hanging in my house; and I would feed him and listen to his troubles. When he met a new lady and she agreed to marry him, he asked me to be his best man. Her grandmother was scandalised at the idea of a woman being a best man and told anyone who would listen that I was a lesbian. When I met her at the kitchen tea and she asked me who I was, I told her I was the lesbian best man. She nearly swallowed her teeth in shock. Sometimes I can be very naughty, but I have a very low tolerance for bigotry.

They had a destination wedding and we all headed off the day before to dress the venue and make all the last-minute preparations. My daughter was going along to oversee the setting up of the venue, while the rest of us were having photographs done. She had a broken hand, but we don't let small things like that get in the way of what needs doing. We are made of much sterner stuff than that. We all piled into bed after dinner. My daughter and I shared a room and we were in a cottage with the groom. I got up to go to the loo in the middle of the night and without warning, I found myself on the bathroom floor, unable to stand. I had an excruciating pain in my right side and I honestly could not stand. I dragged myself along the floor, trying to be quiet so I wouldn't wake the groom. Fortunately, my daughter heard me tapping on our door and she helped me into bed. She phoned her father who, after some pertinent questions were answered, diagnosed kidney stones and recommended that we beat a hasty retreat to the nearest hospital, about an hour's drive away.

Well that wasn't going to happen. I was determined not to ruin the wedding. I set about drinking four litres of water. My daughter, who is also a big fan of the weird shit, did energy healing on me and miraculously, as the sun peeped over the horizon, the stone must have shifted just enough for me to be able to cope. The bride and groom knew nothing of the night's adventures. I cooked us all breakfast, we dressed up in our finery and had all our photographs taken. The wedding went off without a hitch. My daughter fed me paracetamol with a big glass of water every time she went past me and, as the master of ceremonies, I coordinated the reception, including my own speech without mishap. After a couple of dances, my daughter and I slipped away quietly. I was in agony, but as they say in theatrical circles, the show must go on.

Once back in town, I went for a CT scan and that was when I discovered that I had actually broken my back in the Humpty Dumpty fall. I felt pretty vindicated, because I had terrible back pain which, everyone assured me, was because I was overweight. Well it certainly didn't help, but I now knew where it had originated from. I also had a couple of tiny kidney stones. I was cautioned to drink lots of water and wait for them to pass. I bundled along quite happily toting my stones, until one day when I was taking a friend out for breakfast. One minute we were laughing and chatting and the next, I was suddenly felled by a severe pain. This time is was my left side.

I began vomiting and was in a bad way. I had to get to my daughter's house who, fortunately was quite close to where we were. I needed her to drive my friend home and take me to the emergency room. This time the scan showed a massive two-centimetre stone had crashed into the head of my ureter. This required emergency surgery to put in a stent that would protect the kidney and widen the ureter, so that in a separate operation ten days later, the boulder could be blasted and broken up, and the debris removed.

Unfortunately for me, I am allergic to opioids. I'd had a couple of bad experiences with visual and auditory hallucinations and extreme dizziness and confusion after taking pain meds, so I had been warned to stay off all opioids. No one wants to go through kidney stones on paracetamol, but tough Tallulah, I had no choice. It was brutal, but a girl's got to do what a girl's got to do, and somehow, I got through it.

Next up was the cataract debacle. I couldn't see at night, was often experiencing double vision and was battling to read. I trundled off to the eye doctor and was told I had the eyes of an eighty-seven-year old woman. I had cataracts on both eyes. The first one was operated on and the procedure was straight forward. Afterwards however, was a different matter altogether. My brain simply could not deal with the extreme difference in sight between my new lens and the cataract ridden eye. I lost all depth perception, I crashed into walls. If I reached for something, it was never where my hand ended up, I couldn't read, I couldn't watch television and I had flashing white lights in my new good eye.

I went into a state of absolute panic. Since I couldn't drive, my daughter took me back to the eye doctor to discuss this with him. I was terrified of having the second eye done. I was convinced I would go blind. I had lost so much already and was so compromised, I couldn't countenance losing anything more. When I explained what was happening to me, he laughed at me. I'm afraid I didn't see what was funny at all. He hadn't bothered to explain about the transient side effects one can have (I had them all); and in the face of my terror he thought it was funny. I told him I couldn't let him do the second eye and he said fine.

I checked in with my daughter that I hadn't been rude or difficult and she said no, I had been surprisingly well behaved given his response to me in the face of my obvious distress. She thought he'd behaved very badly. That evening he phoned ex-Husband and apologised to him for treating me with less than appropriate professionalism and asked him to convince me to have the second eye done. Why was he apologising to ex-Husband? He hadn't been at the consultation. No one had dismissed him and treated him badly. It must have been that blasted invisibility thing again.

A good friend had in the interim, researched the cataract procedure and explained to me all about the side effects, what could happen and how long they might last. Once I understood it all, I stopped panicking. All of this could have been prevented if only the doctor had treated me with a modicum of decency. Surely it is the doctor's job to reassure and inform the patient? I had the other eye done and now I have really great long-distance vision; and I curse every time I need to find glasses to read anything up close.

Then I had to have my teeth done. All of the above can be attributed to years and years on cortisone. Kidney stones, cataracts, brittle teeth, osteopenia in my spine. That little nugget didn't escape me and I can assure you I was not happy. I had to have fourteen teeth worked on. Amalgam fillings replaced with white fillings, broken teeth capped and two that were beyond repair, removed. It was all done over four appointments. I managed just fine except the fourth anaesthetic sent me into a shock like state. My arms and legs became freezing cold and I shivered uncontrollably. I managed to get home and climbed into bed. In the middle of summer, with hot water bottles and an electric blanket on, it took four hours before warmth began to flow into my arms and legs again and I stopped shaking. It was a most peculiar occurrence.

The dentist said she had never experienced it before. Perhaps it had something to do with the adrenalin in the anaesthetic.

Since I was going through such a tumultuous time with my health, I decided to start looking for a diagnosis again that could explain my situation. I seemed to spend six months researching something, then three to six months trying out a treatment. When I didn't get any relief, I moved on to the next option. I was fast running out of places to look. I decided that in order to cover all the bases on my journey, I owed it to myself to investigate the food is your problem situation. Almost everyone I knew had decided that what I ate was the cause of all my problems and if I was only much slimmer, I would have no issues at all.

The fact that I was relatively slim when all this nonsense started, completely escaped their prejudice. All that notwithstanding I decided to do my due diligence. I had previously gone sugar-free for three months, gluten-free for three months, and dairy free for three months. I tried every diet I could get my hands on and nothing made the slightest bit of difference. In my thirties I had been able to shift weight, but by the time I turned forty it was game over. However, popular opinion always landed on the weight square so, off to a dietician I went. The dietician ran something called nutrigenetic testing. She would have my DNA analysed and would tell me what the optimal eating plan and lifestyle was for my body. That sounded fantastic. Go right to the source of the issue and come out with irrefutable scientifically proven facts. Then design an action plan to correct everything that was wrong with me.

Apparently, I had some slight methylation problems which meant I didn't assimilate nutrients correctly. Also, I would do extremely well as a vegan runner, who slept eight hours a day. Well anyone who knows me, knows that one of my life goals is to run nowhere ever. I can barely bring myself to run to the loo. In fact, I would go so far as to say, if an axe murderer was after me, I would probably lie down and say, "Have at it", rather than run away. So that wasn't going to happen. Besides which, walking was a challenge so running was just not on the cards. Sleeping eight hours a day wasn't an option either because of the sleep apnoea. Ironically if I could get the weight off, the apnoea might resolve, but in order to get the weight off, I needed to sleep. Hmm! Okay so that left me the vegan diet.

I went and walked around the stores and made myself look at the beautifully coloured fruits and vegetables and worked on developing a positive attitude about them. Then I went to the butchery and tortured myself with images of slaughterhouses. I successfully reprogrammed my mind in accordance with my goal. I then booked myself into a health farm and spent three nights in absolute luxury, being massaged and pampered whilst I enjoyed their delicious five-star vegan fare. Mind transformation complete, I followed a strict vegan eating plan for four months. My blood sugar went through the roof, my liver enzymes sky-rocketed, my belly became bloated and so badly swollen that my skin looked silver it was stretched so tight. None of my clothes fit me and I had incredible belly pain. The dietician said she had no idea what to do with me and suggested I go back to my old eating plan and take a month off. We could regroup in the new year and try again. Well you can imagine how I heard that suggestion. I did stop the vegan diet, but my belly became more and more painful. I had to buy clothes two sizes larger to fit them over my distended bump.

I visited a general surgeon who performed colonoscopies and told him about my very sad belly. He did an examination and said, "There is nothing wrong with your belly. However, since you are over fifty and you've never had a colonoscopy, perhaps we should schedule one just to be thorough." I had just changed medical aids and there was a three month wait on procedures. I was assured again there was nothing wrong and I was fine to wait. So, I took my distended, painful, apparently perfectly healthy belly and I left. I was in hell.

One day I drove past a spiritualist church and they were advertising an open day. I stopped and went inside. My senses were assaulted by so much incense. Every stall holder seemed to be burning some and the smell was overwhelming. There was woo-woo music playing in the background and all around the room, people were sitting or lying down and someone was doing hands on healing on them. There were tarot readers, psychics, crystal readers and many things I had never heard of. I walked past a table and an Indian lady called to me to sit down. She looked at me with so much kindness and she said, "You are in so much pain and yet you smile. How are you managing to do this?"

"You have a terrible pain in your belly and you need urgent medical attention. This is very serious." I sat there and the tears poured down my face. Finally, someone could see me as I truly was. It was such a relief to admit that, yes, I was in agony and even though doctors and specialists had told me there was nothing wrong with me, I was in fact feeling so ill I didn't know how to keep going. I agreed to schedule the colonoscopy as soon as possible, medical aid be damned. That is what credit cards are for in my life, emergencies.

Since I was there, I signed up for a Reiki treatment and had myself ironed. That lady was also terribly kind and kept telling me how worried she was about me and that I must take care of myself. Then I went to see a psychic. He looked like a regular chap, no frills and paraphernalia. I waited my turn and when he invited me to sit at his table, he immediately said, "I have two gentlemen stepping forward." I looked around to see if I had, by mistake, jumped the queue. He laughed and said that they were stepping forward for me. Aha! He was a medium and folk in Spirit wanted to talk to me.

He positioned the two men as an older gentleman, perhaps my father and the other man who was family but not family. My sister and her partner had never married and I asked him, "Is this my sister's partner?" Turned out it was. He chatted with me through the psychic for almost an hour. He spoke about how much he had loved my sister and he said it was time for him to leave because he had done everything he needed to do. He had needed me to be there for her so that he could leave.

He said things like, "Life is short, eat the chocolate cake, you know you want to." This was something he and my sister used to argue about. He had a terribly sweet tooth and loved chocolate cake. She always told him he couldn't have any and so every time he went into town, he would sneak himself a slice of guilt-free cake. Having me there to stay he had support for his cake fetish. He always used to say, "Have a piece of cake Jan, life's too short, you know you want to," and he would join me. He spoke about his love of fishing and alluded to one night when we had eaten our body weight in garlic prawns.

There were so many references that were private and no one could possibly have known about, that I was in no doubt I was indeed communicating with him. He spoke about my Warthog Tales book and said that I would be writing another book that would also be very successful. It had something to do with the energy stuff I had been working on. I had just finished editing the Inner Tuition manual. It was such a joy to hear from him and to know that he was happy. He assured me that there was still so much life ahead for my sister, if she could only allow herself to reach for it.

I was having a particularly bad night, I had so much pain and bloating. I was sweating and shaking, I was terribly worried. I called on the group of Inner Tuition energy healers once again. They are a wonderful bunch of incredibly gifted and generous healers and if anyone ever asked for help or called for support for someone they knew who was in crisis, there was always at least one of us who would answer the call. These were the ladies I had called on when my sister's partner had passed away, also when my daughter was car-jacked. Since energy healing can be done remotely, we are able to tap into the person's energy field and assist as needed, always with a prayer of protection and asking permission from both our, and their Spirit Guides.

I received so many urgent messages that night telling me I was in the throes of a life-threatening crisis. They worked furiously to untangle my colon and to send energy through to parts that were dying. This gave me the final push I needed and I went in for my colonoscopy. It was performed under conscious sedation and because of my opioid sensitivity I couldn't have the pain relief. I figured that I had managed the kidney stones, so this should be a walk in the park.

Well, I was completely oblivious, but they ended up abandoning the procedure after completing only one third of the colon. I apparently screamed in such agony that people were coming up from the next floor of the building to see who was being murdered. They removed quite a few polyps from the short segment and also found diverticulosis. One section of my colon was twisted on itself and was in danger of dying off. If I had waited the three months for the medical aid to kick in, I would have been having a portion of my colon removed and would have ended up with a temporary colostomy bag. I was requested to book myself in for the remainder of the procedure to be done under general anaesthetic. Score one for the weird shit folk and bah humbug to the bloody doctors who appear to know nothing, certainly when it comes to my health.

Life Lessons:

- There truly is no end to the awfulness that is my health
- I am one tough cookie
- I am dependable no matter what it costs me
- The doctors simply cannot see me
- Somehow Spirit seems to be watching out for me
- A soul who passes over into Spirit can communicate with you

Chapter 32

The teaching conundrum

It was time for me to teach an Inner Tuition course. I had attended so many by now, acting as co-facilitator for a few of them and my friend was looking for someone else to take over the teaching role. I was really excited about this opportunity and I could see so much overlap with what I had learned in the corporate world and what I had learned from Inner Tuition. I was eager to share this all with the students. It proved a difficult exercise however, not because I couldn't teach the work, but because my friend really wasn't ready to let go control.

It was a tremendous learning experience for me to see her struggle and to realise that her behaviour in no way reflected on my capability, it was about her struggle with relinquishing her life's work to another. I finally learned to recognise when something was about me and more importantly, when it wasn't. We always say that everything is exactly as it should be and even if we cannot understand the reason why things happen, we are to trust that it is all scripted and a higher purpose is being served. This proved very true when I ended up with a catastrophic injury that necessitated her having to take over the teaching role mid-course. This worked out rather well in fact. My friend happily took over the reins again and I could finally start to do the work on myself that I had been too afraid to do for the past twenty odd years.

I had been sitting cross legged on my bedroom floor painting my chest of drawers. I had done everything back to front, but I was too sore to keep getting up and then down again. Sitting on the floor was a painful exercise. So, when I realised that I needed to take out the heavy drawers to paint properly, I did just that. Sitting on the ground I lifted a heavy drawer above my head, twisted right around to put it on the bed behind me and something went snap! It was down the side of my trunk on the right-hand side towards the front and it was excruciating. Sweat poured down my back and I was panting in pain. I couldn't get up, I couldn't get down, my legs had gone completely dead and I was well and truly stuck. After a long while realising there was nothing I could do, I concentrated hard on moving the pain to the back of my mind and I finished painting what I could reach on the chest of drawers.

A couple of hours later, ex-Husband came home and helped me up onto my bed. I was in trouble. It was the start of a long weekend and I couldn't get to anyone for help. My first thought was to get to my trusty chiropractor, but he was away for the four-day weekend. I was given an anti-inflammatory injection and put to bed. And that's where I stayed. Once again, all alone in a sea of pain, with no help at hand, no idea what was wrong and no solutions. The most I could manage was to shuffle along the wall to the bathroom.

I couldn't stand long enough to fill a water bottle without crying in pain. I decided to try something new. I googled physiotherapists in my area who did house calls. There was no way I could get to anyone, so I needed someone to come to me. I was incredibly lucky to find an amazing lady who not only knew her craft extremely well, she also understood a lot about weird shit. We clicked right from the start. The day she arrived I had developed a sudden onset migraine headache. I hadn't had one of those since I left the office.

She arrived to find me hunched miserably over the toilet bowl, vomiting. Not a problem, she helped me onto her massage bed and began to rub a spot on the front of my neck. As if by magic the migraine and the nausea dissolved and it was as though it had never happened. She diagnosed me with a catastrophic psoas muscle injury. She went on to explain that psoas was a rather tricky muscle. It held one upright and propelled one forward. It was also well connected with matters of childhood trauma and feelings of being unsafe. My psoas had a lot to say and it was screaming at the top of its lungs. She visited me at home twice a week for about two months before I was well enough to drive to her studio. It's almost two years later and I still see her weekly. She has learned to hear my body when it talks and she knows just how to talk back so that it responds.

That was how I found myself lying on a couch at the Inner Tuition course, having students practice their craft on me. No longer teaching and largely incapacitated, I was perfectly positioned to start working on those inner child issues. That was what my psoas muscle injury seemed to be telling me to do, so… As they delved into my chakras and my inner child memories they picked-up bits and pieces of my childhood trauma. I began to process the information and to allow myself to look at it through adult eyes. I understood for the first time what I had gone through and I was able, through meditation, to go back as an adult version of myself and rescue those parts of me that had gotten stuck. I'll explain this a little clearer in section three. I was starting to find my power and to connect with my full potential.

Feeling much better about myself than I had in months, I had gone to a friend's home where her son was having a birthday party. There were crowds of lanky nineteen-year olds all speaking a foreign form of English. The generation gap created a barrier that truly prevented me from understanding most of what they said, plus they spoke too fast for my ringing ears to translate. We were chatting round the fire when suddenly there was a commotion. Turned out one of the boys' younger brother had snuck in some drugs which he had taken and he was having a really bad reaction.

When we got to him, he was having a full-blown tonic clonic seizure. We flipped him into recovery position and called the paramedics. They seemed to take forever to arrive. As he postured and seized, I couldn't stand to watch. Throwing all fear of being seen as a person who dabbles in weird shit to the wind, I got down on the floor with him and muttering a prayer of protection, I invoked every Spirit Guide and helper from Upstairs I could think of to assist. I put my hands into his energy field. Over and over I muttered, "Let that which is for the highest good of all concerned manifest for this child."

It isn't for me to know what was right for this boy and far be it for me to interfere in something he needed to go through, but I needed to do something and by invoking his highest good, I was removing myself from the equation and was simply connecting him with his Spirit Guides asking for their help. The seizure moved from his body right into mine. I felt it go up my arms. My muscles spasmed and pulled tight and then it travelled upwards and was released through the top of my head. The beautiful, stupid young man lay still and quiet and as he relaxed, he began to regain consciousness. By the time the paramedics arrived he was sitting up protesting how fine he was and his mother, who had arrived just ahead of them, agreed not to send him to hospital. If she had arrived a few minutes sooner and seen him in the state he was in, I doubt she would have been so accommodating. The paramedics shook their heads and made her sign a form to say she was acting against their advice. She went home, the music started up again and the party carried on.

I was horrified, not only by what had happened to this child, but at how unaffected the youngsters were. One of their own had had a full-blown seizure on the floor and it was over as though it had never happened. I am so afraid for this next generation. They seem to think they are Teflon coated and nothing can stick to them. Somehow, they would always get to have a do over, or a reset. Nothing ever seems to be their fault, and they take little or no responsibility for their choices. This leaves them so vulnerable and distances them from their humanity. It's almost as though their moral compasses appear to be on the fritz. I do believe that if I hadn't been allowed to pull that seizure from that child's body, that evening may well have ended much more tragically. I understood in that moment, the importance of reclaiming my damaged inner child so that I might help other youngsters in life.

Life Lessons:

- Adversity can sometimes be a blessing in disguise
- It isn't all about me
- With hard work, it is possible to reclaim and heal parts of you that are wounded
- Teenagers are a troubled bunch
- Drugs are dangerous
- I have work to do

Chapter 33

The depression conundrum

At this junction, life is still happening to me. I feel as though I have no part to play in my own destiny as I sit and wait for the next blow, the next disaster, the next loss. I have realised that I have so much to offer and I yearn to feel useful and functional again, yet I struggle to find the courage of my convictions. I feel as though I am living two lives at the same time. One very much a victim of circumstance, unworthy, disallowed, unempowered, physically challenged; the other bursting with potential, powerful, filled with hope and possibility. Yet, still I feel frozen, unable to move forward not only because of my physical limitations, but largely because I feel tethered by my past. The loudest voice in my mind that still makes the final decision for me, is Mother's. I have no value, no worth. People like me can expect nothing from life. Who do I think I am?

It had been suggested to me by almost every medical doctor I had consulted (and by this stage there had been many), that I was suffering from depression and everything else flowed from there. My symptoms were all psychosomatic and there really wasn't anything wrong with me. I decided it might be time to go down that rabbit hole and do my due diligence, as I did with all diagnoses that were suggested to me. After the great lupus conundrum, I was no longer prepared to accept anything from a doctor without doing my own research and determining for myself if the diagnosis was correct.

I consulted a clinical psychologist to discuss my depression. We had four or five sessions together before she said the following to me, "You have to be the least depressed person I have ever met. You meet none of the criteria for any form of depression. You, however, are quite the saddest person I have ever met and with very good reason." I was ecstatic to finally be able to put the depression conundrum to rest. I thanked her profusely and went off to digest this nugget of information.

I was surprised to discover that I had no idea I was so sad. I identified my emotions as anger, frustration, disappointment and remorse. I hadn't really considered sadness. I realised that the picklist of emotions I allowed myself to select from was so limited as to be a problem in itself. I wonder how many other people are walking around with the erroneous thinking that they are depressed, anxious or angry, when in fact they are experiencing something else entirely and they simply do not have the emotional vocabulary to identify with. I decided to take a long hard look at emotions.

I looked up the term emotional intelligence and it is defined as the capacity to be aware of, control, and express one's emotions, and to handle interpersonal relationships judiciously and empathetically. This definition was followed up with this sweeping statement: emotional intelligence is the key to both personal and professional success. There are five components to emotional intelligence, being self-awareness, self-management, motivation, empathy and social skills. Clearly, I was a bit of an emotional underachiever. This surprised me because I understood implicitly that I was ruled by my emotions. After a good long look, I realised that whilst I was highly motivated, I was empathetic to the point of self-destruction. I attributed this to an inherent lack of self-awareness and self-management which had an adverse effect on my social skills. All those years of hiding out, of being seen and not heard, of speaking only when spoken to, of not being allowed to be who I truly felt I was inside, had resulted in me growing into a veritable emotional cripple.

Through this crippling inability to properly identify and manage my emotions, I had allowed myself to be bullied, silenced, ignored, manipulated, used, moulded, altered, diminished, labelled and dismissed to the point where I was frozen in fear; fear of becoming who I yearned to be, and fear of staying the same. I needed a crash course in emotions and I needed it fast. If I was to start on a journey of self-discovery and liberation from my past then I needed to learn the language of emotions. I read a great article detailing the signs of a high EQ (emotional intelligence) and I decided to take a moment of honest reflection.

- You have a robust emotional vocabulary – clearly, I did not meet that criteria
- You're curious about people – I'm terrified of people I don't know, and hide from the ones I do
- You embrace change – this one I am surprisingly good with, but I guess if your situation is bad enough then change is the only way out so you learn to be nimble
- You know your strengths and weaknesses – this one was a real challenge because I was never sure which me I was thinking about; the outer me being the angry warrior with a world sized

chip on her shoulder, or the inner powerful me who could take charge and make a difference in the world

- You're a good judge of character – I think I'm pretty good with this. Ever heard the saying don't try to bullshit a bullshitter? I can spot a bad guy or a pretender from a mile away.
- You are difficult to offend – I can be offended by the way people blink when in my company. I read censure and judgement in the tilt of a head, and the tone of a voice can send me into a complete tailspin
- You know how to say no (to yourself and others) – One of my life's goals is to learn to say no and I remain stubbornly optimistic that one day I shall acquire this great skill
- You let go of mistakes – nope sorry, I hang onto every transgression. I learned that from the cradle courtesy of *them*.

There are so many articles and books available on the subject of emotional health and how you can become stronger emotionally. As usual the cliff notes version I took away was as follows:

There are six basic human emotions: happiness, sadness, fear, anger, surprise and disgust. There are myriad emotional offshoots of these six. Emotions are felt in the body as physical sensations. I had never made that connection before and I was fascinated. Once you can connect the physical feeling with each of these emotions you can begin to adjust your behaviour to support a healthier emotional state.

Having finally made the mind body connection, it became apparent to me that the multitude of mystery symptoms I was experiencing could well be either as a direct result of repressed emotions, or at the very least they could be exacerbating a physiological condition. Medicine didn't appear to have the answers for me. I knew I wasn't clinically depressed. What to do? I realised I could either spend the rest of my days ruled by the emotions of fear and sadness or I could begin the deep dive journey work required to bring myself into the light. I had come across these concepts during my flirtations with the all the weird shit I had encountered. Fear was the overriding reason that I had run away from each encounter. It was time to take charge of life instead of waiting to see what it would dish out to me. It was time to fully embrace the weird shit and get to work!

Have a look at Plutchick's Wheel of Emotion on the next page.

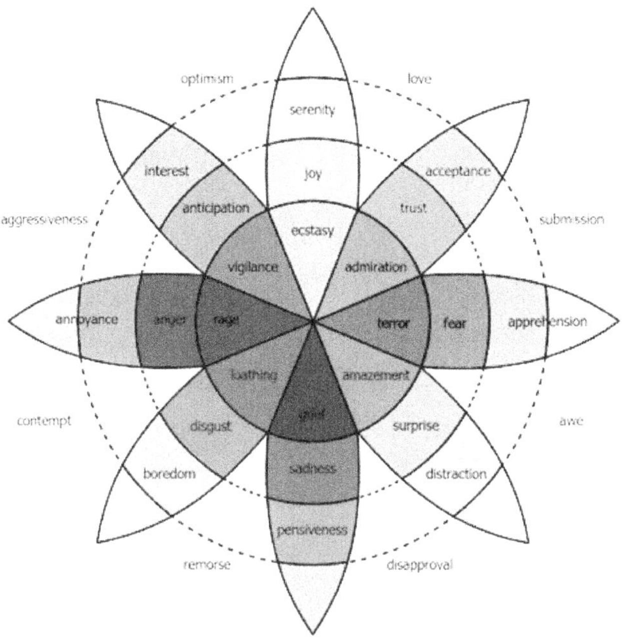

Life lessons:

- Nothing amazing ever happens in your comfort zone
- You truly have nothing to fear, but fear itself
- Nothing changes, until you change it.
- I am the master of my own destiny (well I really hope I am)

Part Three

The weird shit explained

Chapter 34

A general philosophy

I have learned so much from so many different sources and when you break it all down to the simplest components, almost all of them are saying exactly the same thing. They use different language and they coin different catch phrases, but in reality, it is all the same. Pretty much as it is with religion, where each group believes in a higher power, there are rules and regulations, there are places of worship and people to guide and watch over the masses. There are punishments for incorrect behaviour, and of course the ultimate reward at the end of life is to be admitted into that place where the higher power resides. You will thus be blessed with eternal life.

Obviously, there are variations on that theme, but when one strips it right back to the bare bones, the matrix is really the same. I am constantly perplexed therefore, how each different group believes in their innate rightness to the total exclusion of all other groups. If they all believe they are right, then how on earth are we to know who actually is? Right there, is where the world of Energy / Spirit / Upstairs / Universe (call it what you will), coincides with organised religion. They are all right. I don't believe they are managed very well though, because they seem to stop short of giving their followers that final piece of the puzzle, the ability to attain enlightenment without anyone, be it a deity or figurehead, having to intercede on their behalf.

To do so would mean losing control over them and as with all large controlling bodies that are primarily businesses, religions are indeed controlling. The world of energy can be like that too and many practices are heavily influenced by the ego of the practitioners. However, pure energy work, done with absolute integrity, has no place for the ego. It is about equipping people with tools and skills so that they are able to do their own work and heal their own wounds. No one can heal another person and one should be very wary of any practitioner who claims to be able to do so.

The philosophy I have adopted is quite simple really. We are not humans seeking spiritual enlightenment through the intercession of a deity, but rather we are spiritual beings, having a human experience, through the medium of love. This is a critical distinction and bears repeating. *We are spiritual beings, having a human experience, through the medium of love.* We are already whole and in fact, we are Universal love, we are the One. There is no need to atone for anything to become AT-ONE with all that is, (see how that word takes on a whole new meaning with a slight shift in perspective).

We are already at one with the light, we have simply forgotten how to shine. Now, when I say through the medium of love, please understand that is an all-encompassing expression for all aspects of love; the fullness of love, the absence of love, the seeking of love, the denying of love, the disillusionment of love; and so on ad infinitum. There can be no denying the existence of a greater power, although many will tell you, through their own disillusion, that there is none.

We are all here on this Earth as humans and we all suffer from afflictions of love in one form or another. We drive ourselves to the point of insanity trying to find love, or we deny our right to be loved and drive ourselves to the edges of despair. The permutations of love are almost infinite. If we are loved too well, we might become spoiled, pampered, or perhaps entitled; if we are not loved enough, we become wounded, fearful and sometimes bitter. Either way our reality gets distorted. We need to learn to simply *be* without judgement or prejudice.

We hear a lot from our political and religious leaders about how we should practice tolerance. Humans seem to have a built-in fear of anything that is beyond their ken, different from them. We hold everything we encounter up against the framework of our life experiences and the doctrines we have been taught. If there isn't a match, we determine to keep that which is different from us outside of our experience. This leads to separateness and creates more distortions of love. If we allow for the possibility that a different point of view or perspective has any real merit, then our beliefs and our reality come under threat. Everything on planet Earth is governed by duality. In or out, right or wrong, up or down, good or bad, black or white, gay or straight... the list goes on. In a binary world there is little accommodation for the middle ground.

So many interactions between people and groups seem to be about one side trying to convince the other side that their ways, views, behaviours and morals are the only way and any deviation from that makes the other person somehow less than or inferior. They become someone to be kept firmly on the outside, or they are at best magnanimously tolerated. I find the word tolerance to be one of the most offensive words in the English language.

How dare you presume to tolerate me. What gives you the upper hand and the right to tolerate me, with the inference being that your way is somehow superior to mine and I am somehow less than you are because of our differences. Some of the most interesting people I know are those with whom I have absolutely nothing in common. I love listening to how they think and what motivates them and to see the conclusions they draw about the world at large.

If nothing else, those interactions open my mind to perspectives I may never have known about. I would never dare to presume to tolerate their views. I accept them with an open heart, with respect for the fact that they are the beliefs of another soul. What we seem to fail miserably at, is grasping the concept that we do not have to agree on a single thing, to be kind to one another. I would never presume to tell someone that their beliefs are wrong and then make myself seem to be a better person by tolerating them.

In my humble opinion one of the greatest distortions of love in our world today is this notion of tolerance. It is one of the primary reasons why humanity is in such a state right now. Fear has taken over our planet and people are clustered together in the safety of their like-minded groups, clutching onto their beliefs and the safety of their taught doctrines, steadfastly excluding and keeping out anything that even comes close to being different. If only we could learn to appreciate one another and to celebrate our differences, what a very different existence we would have.

I believe that our job on this earth is to effect our own healing and to find love within ourselves. Whether we use Christ Jesus as the medium for that healing, or the great Buddha, or Allah, or any other recognisable deity, or whether we battle it out in the wilderness on our own, our mission remains the same, to find that pure love inside of ourselves. We are all aspects of the greater Universe that seeks to express itself in every possible permutation. If the Universe at large is the expression of all that is and defines itself as the purest form of love and light, then our function as spiritual beings, is to explore humanity in all its various guises and to master each aspect of it. By doing so we become whole.

We are taught that we are made in His images. Well stripped down to the bare bones, that is exactly what I am saying. The way to true enlightenment and to attain that place on high is to completely master every single aspect of being human. That explains why some folk appear to be more highly evolved than others, they have been at it longer and have mastered more aspects. Because we have this wonderful thing called free will on our planet, it is too easy to go off track and it can sometimes take us a long time to master any one particular aspect. Let me explain how I think this all goes down.

Firstly, I believe that we have many, many lifetimes to explore our humanity. The task is simply too great to be accomplished in one go. A lot of religions hold the single lifetime scenario over the heads of their followers to ensure compliance with the rules. If you know you get do overs then why would you follow the rules. If you don't get it right there is a figurehead or deity who can and will intercede on your behalf, so either way you are pretty much taken care of.

The missing link for me with religion is that it doesn't allow for personal accountability. There is no imperative to figure things out your own way, just follow the yellow brick road, join the dots, do as you are taught and eternity shall be yours. The entirety of the extent of the Universe is simply beyond anything the human brain can imagine or encompass. Therefore, religious texts are simplified to make them more easily understandable. I believe however, that they are not the final word, but an interpretation of something too vast to portray.

Imagine if you will, the *big guy in the sky* (being representative of all that is) as a five-thousand-piece jigsaw puzzle. The completed picture will be Him in all His glory, made visible for us, the mere mortals. Remembering that we are created in His image, so it is incumbent upon us to find all the puzzle pieces and work out how to fit them all together. By doing so we may finally see that which we so longingly seek. The scope and vastness of this great puzzle is too great for our brains to countenance so we need to approach it a little a time.

We can build ourselves up to the point where finally, the scales fall from our eyes and we truly see. We stand in all our glory and full technicolour splendour and we become a part of all that is, that ultimate reward for a life well lived. There are thousands of pieces of that puzzle to be identified and correctly positioned before we can see the full picture. Each aspect of humanity is one of the pieces. Let's assume for the sake of an example that one of the pieces is abandonment. I might design myself a lifetime that includes contracts with members of my soul group who agree to be the people who will abandon me thus allowing me to have this experience.

Having found that puzzle piece, I still do not know where to place it, because there is more to it. I might therefore design a second lifetime where I am the one to do the abandoning. I will add a cast of characters who agree to be wounded by my abandonment of them and I can explore the other side of this aspect. Once I have all aspects of abandonment mastered, I can place my puzzle piece and go on to find the next piece. With each piece I add, the image becomes clearer until finally I have the full picture. This is the way to enlightenment, through self-exploration. Until we master all aspects of ourselves and realise that we were perfect all along and we are in fact already divine, we will keep on seeking.

The confounding thing about life here as a human on planet Earth, is that we exist at such a low vibrational frequency, we lose a lot of our clarity just by being here. Quick interjection here of a science experiment every school going child on the planet has been exposed to. Everything is energy. Energy cannot be destroyed; it can only be transformed (changed from one form to another). Take a solid ice block and stress it by adding heat. The molecules in the ice begin to vibrate at a different frequency and the ice is transformed into water. Exactly the same energy, just moving faster. By continually adding more pressure in the form of more heat, the water evaporates. It begins moving at such a high frequency one can almost not see it with the naked eye as it is transformed into steam. So, with the understanding that everything is energy and energy can only be transformed and not destroyed, imagine if you will that you are a divine spiritual being (energy) with something you need to master.

- Having chosen the lesson, path, goal or objective for this incarnation, you set about creating a life plan or a project plan if you will. This is a complicated plan that has to allow for all and any eventuality. Remember we have free will and are therefore prone to wandering off course. Contingencies must be built in. I will explain more about this.
- You've appointed your Spirit Guides. These are your silent partners who can assist only when specifically asked and may not get involved in the day to day running of your life.
- You have signed on guardian angels to protect you from yourself, because, having been to Earth before, you know how easy it is to go astray. One wrong left turn and you can find yourself in a heap of trouble. This is where these guys come in extremely handy. I like to think of them as the sweepers in the sport of curling. They work furiously to remove dangers and obstacles from your path.
- You have cast members from your soul group to play your parents, siblings, teachers, pupils, protagonists, demons, drivers, supporters and oh so much more. It is really a complex thing planning a life. This is a good place to hook in with souls who may need to master the other side of your particular mission. A soul who was a thief in their last lifetime may need to come back and experience being a victim of crime to fully understand and

master the entire aspect. Your life plan may involve some skull-duggery and you can therefore dovetail your plans.

- You build in all the criteria needed for your incoming soul to exist on Earth; birth circumstances, country, racial profile, sexual preference, carers, parents, peer group, community groups, all aspects of your childhood, adolescence, adulthood, friends, foes, teachers, followers, health issues, accidents and trauma, the whole nine yards. Remember all the contingency plans too. All of this has the purpose of helping you to find that aspect of yourself which you are incarnating to master.
- Your Higher Self, that part of you that knows everything about you already, including the bits you still need to find out about, will act as project manager. They are there for you to check in with, should you need to regroup along the way (just as soon as you remember that they exist of course).
- You also put in an entire cheering section. These are souls who have chosen not to incarnate at that time, perhaps they are taking a sabbatical from self-mastery and prefer to sit this round out, or perhaps they have found all their puzzle pieces. They are however, as part of your soul group, vastly interested in your progress and will be cheering you on since there is a no man left behind policy in soul groups. Each group needs to have all its members reach the same level of enlightenment, before they can graduate to a different area of work in the universe, it is therefore critical that they support and assist in your quest. Once total humanity is achieved, souls can become guardians of animals, or nature, or custodians of the greater cosmos. The vastness of the possibilities is, remember, beyond our comprehension.
- Launch birth plan. This involves slowing down your vibration to the almost unbearably dense vibration of human life. You press Go on the game board and your contracted characters begin to play out the scenarios that will ultimately lead to your conception. I always think of the sci-fi epic "Beam me up Scotty", except you are being beamed down. Once your host (mother), becomes aware that you are there, you can begin to assimilate information. Is she pleased that you are there, does she want you to be born, is she fearful, were the circumstances around your conception ideal or perhaps traumatic, does she take care of her health giving you optimum growing conditions…? You continue growing in the human way and, assuming your life plan involved you being birthed as a healthy human baby, you go through the traumatic experience of being born. All the while you

were growing in utero, you were assimilating information from your mother's body, but at the same time you were losing clarity on the life plan you created. It is terribly hard to retain that amount of information at this new, more dense vibration. Then once you experience the trauma of birth (and I can attest here, having gone through mine again with the hairy therapist, that it is not a comfortable process), the trauma wipes the last connection with your plan from your mind. You no longer have a clue why you have arrived here helpless and confused, and you begin your lifelong search for the answers to the questions, "Who am I?" and "Why am I here?"

Chapter 35

Some terminology explained

Again, drawing from myriad sources, I shall attempt to explain certain concepts, terms and words that I shall be using. You may or may not have come across them already, which is fine. If everything is new to you, you may decide I am a total nut job and move on with your ordinary life, no harm, no foul; or you may be intrigued and continue reading, which will delight me no end. If some, or all of this, is already familiar, well that is just wonderful. If my description of something is at odds with your understanding, that too is well and good.

When I did my psychic development workshops, the facilitator assigned different colours to each of the chakras than I was used to. This confronted me no end until I understood that it worked for her and she was teaching me her interpretation of chakras. I had no right to expect her to conform to popular opinion. I was there to learn from her and so learn from her I would. I would later make my own decisions about how chakras were to be represented in my life. Free will people, free will.

Upstairs

Right, for the purposes of brevity and copying shamelessly from Inner Tuition (with kind permission, I hasten to add), I shall refer to anything beyond the pale of the earthly sphere as Upstairs. This wonderful collective term simplifies the process of writing and understanding really well and also helps to sidestep the zealots who are firmly attached to their particular terminology.

This term includes, but is not limited to, all recognised deities, God, Buddha, Allah, Angels, Spirit, Spirit Guides, the Universe, Heaven, *the Big Guy in the Sky*, All That Is, the One, the Light, and indeed anything else of that ilk. In a world governed by duality there is *Us* and there is *Them. They* are all lumped under the label of Upstairs and all of us *mere mortals* are referred to as Us. *They* are not to be confused with Mother's auditory hallucinations. That was something else entirely. See how easily one word can hold two meanings. The directive from Upstairs is to achieve the enlightenment of all souls connected with Earth. Other planets may have their own goals, but for those of us connected with Earth, this is our directive.

Soul groups

It is my profound belief that souls travel in groups. For souls, please understand that I am referring to all beings whether in Spirit (Upstairs), or in human form. Soul groups are comprised of many hundreds, maybe even thousands of souls. These soul groups form various collective consciousnesses. What I mean by that is that the evolution of a soul is a complex matter and needs to be handled one bite at a time. Each stage of a soul's evolution forms a group consciousness. If you think of it in terms of how we go through the various stages of being human it gives you a fair understanding of what I mean:

- We start out as *babies* with primal, basic needs, focussed only upon our own survival and our immediate self. We need others to take care of the rules and the responsibilities. There are so many people in the baby soul stage walking this earth who are in this primitive evolutionary stage. They have just begun their soul's journey to enlightenment. They are largely unconcerned with how things are run. They are self-involved or inwardly focussed on their own basic need for safety and survival.
- Then we move on to the *toddler* stage. Here we realise that we are separate from our mothers. We begin to interact with others and understand there are others just like us. We are focussed on acquisition of skills, walking, talking, self-feeding and so on and are working towards becoming independent. Someone in the toddler soul stage might begin to take some responsibility for their own well-being. They still require rules and structure to be taken care of by someone else, but they begin to interact with the world around them, they begin to be useful in society.
- The next phase is the *child* where we are focussed on actively separating from our parents. We learn to think for ourselves and we strive for autonomy, but we still need a strong guiding force. A person with a child soul can become somewhat disruptive as they struggle for independence. They need to learn the rules of society and begin to self-regulate their behaviours.
- Once we hit *adolescence* however, we begin to challenge the teachings and boundaries of our caregivers and authorities. We begin to form strong opinions about who we are as individuals. People in this soul group may well be controversial. They are the

great debaters of the world and they are not those who blindly accept the rules. They need to understand and be convinced before they will align themselves.

- The *youth* phase once again plunges us into an acquisition phase of life. We focus on acquiring higher education or trades that help us identify ourselves in the context of everything else. People in this soul group are very focussed on their own identity. They like to study and learn and are focussed on building something to make their mark. These people identify strongly with their chosen profession or trade.
- As an *adult* we are all about the interaction with others. We acquire status through our chosen profession, we may choose a mate and have children, we begin to influence the world around us. Adult souls are those that seek to expand their existence. They are focussed on community, togetherness and growth. They like to identify with their acquisitions or whatever they perceive to be of value and they seek to effect change in the world.
- Then finally we become *elderly*. With the accumulated wisdom of all of the preceding stages we hold a vast body of knowledge. We are able to see with greater clarity how everything fits together. We begin to focus on the end of the journey. Souls in this stage are the leaders of communities, the elders, the rule setters or the change agents, those who inspire and support the younger souls. They are our philosophers, our writers and our teachers. They are benevolent and no longer invested in ego and focus instead on the bigger picture aspects of life.

If you extrapolate out and think of different people in your lives, or different cultures, or societies, even countries… you can generally see at which stage of evolution that soul, or soul group is. This explains why there are so many variances in the human experience. As with anything in life, one needs to master the basics before progressing to more challenging or complex matters until reaching full understanding.

It is prudent to acknowledge too, that an older person does not castigate a younger child for that which they have not yet been exposed to, learned or mastered. They support and teach and with patience, they foster understanding and growth. There is no expectation of a baby to earn a living. Being angry at a person who is at a lower level of soul evolution is as futile as being angry at a toddler because it can't cook you a gourmet meal or solve a mathematical equation. We waste so much energy focussing on our separateness and differences, when in fact we are all the same, just at varying developmental levels.

Once an entire soul group has attained their particular level of enlightenment, they can progress to the next soul level (life stage). Each soul group requires different guides and helpers who are specialised in each particular level. They are highly evolved souls that take on these roles, think here of Christ, Buddha, the Archangels and so on. Using my corporate life as an analogy, think of each soul group as the equivalent of a department. The big guns as heads of department, or middle management as it were. Each group is responsible for managing, maintaining, balancing their collective part of the whole, or their department as it were. Remember the cosmos at large, is so much more than we can comprehend and so this is of necessity, a much-simplified explanation.

As mentioned, your soul group may include hundreds of souls and you all travel together through multiple incarnations playing differing roles in one another's life plans. Sometimes choosing to not incarnate at all, but to guide from Upstairs. If you ask yourself why, with the millions of people walking this Earth, you only connect with a mere handful, you may begin to understand soul groups. There is a recognition between you that happens on an energetic level to which you are completely unconscious. Your Higher Self will recognise these people as players in your life plan, even if you do not, and as your project manager, they will have engineered meetings and situations for you to connect. Looking back on my life, I can see that anything that had a profound effect on me, I had been made aware of many years before I actually took notice. My project manager has had a tough job with me.

Higher Self

This is your soul's fullest expression of itself. That which is *made in His image* if you like. You are an aspect of *all that is* and you have your own unique colour signature which is the cosmic equivalent of a human fingerprint. Your Higher Self knows everything about you through all your incarnations and is the ultimate goal towards which you, as a human being, are working. Once you have mastered all aspects of your humanity, you can cease your searching and exist as a fully evolved, enlightened soul. It is logical then that project management would fall within this role.

Energy field

We understand and accept that everything is energy vibrating at different frequencies. There is a wonderful technology available called Kirlian photography. Using this method, one is able to see the energy field around an object. One of the more well-known experiments was the torn leaf experiment. A section of a leaf is torn away yet the Kirlian photographs revealed the energy field of the whole leaf. It has been conjectured that this could explain the phantom limb pain often experienced by amputees. They are bombarded by pain and sensation in the area where their amputated limb used to be. Their energy field remembers the whole body and is still reacting to the trauma of the amputation.

There are many different interpretations regarding the human energy field. Based on what I have learned and experienced, I am comfortable stating that there is so much more to us than our physical bodies and that which can be perceived with the naked eye. We have an electromagnetic field around our body, or an *etheric* body if you like. This is made up of four subtle bodies, each vibrating at a different frequency.

So, we have our actual body, the vehicle through which we experience this life, then a *physical* energetic or etheric body, an *emotional* energetic or etheric body, a *mental* energetic or etheric body, and a *spiritual* energetic or etheric body. These four subtle bodies are all contained within our aura.

We also have a system of energy centres running, interconnected, through our body called *chakras*; and a system of meridians through which energy flows to all areas of our body. None of this is visible to the naked eye. There is however, a great deal of information in Indian and Chinese writings describing this in detail. The Aboriginal cultures of Australia are aware of this etheric energy system and use it in their art, music, costume and religious practices.

Within the energy field is stored all the information required by the soul for the incarnation at hand; the blueprints for your current life plan and all relevant information from previous incarnations. We do not immediately know how to connect with these energy fields or how to access this information and that is why so many of us spend decades, if not lifetimes, struggling to find our way.

The analogy I like to use to explain the four etheric bodies is the printing presses. My Dad was a printer and I used to go to the factory with him on the weekends and watch the Smartie boxes running on the machines. It was so exciting to see how everything just ran and flowed and how a blank piece of paper could be overlaid with only four colours and suddenly, as if by magic, an image of Smarties in all of their gorgeous colours would appear.

The four colour plates from which all colours are created on a printing press are cyan, magenta, yellow and finally black. Once the first plate has run with the first colour, the image is laid down on the paper, but as a single colour it remains indistinct. As each subsequent colour is added the image becomes clearer until that grand moment when the final colour, black, is laid down. Suddenly, absolute clarity is achieved and you know exactly what you are looking at. It truly is magical. If, however, one of the printing plates was not properly calibrated and aligned, that colour would have printed slightly out of register and the final image would be fuzzy and unclear.

It's the same with the human body. If one of our bodies is out of balance our lives can become very fuzzy indeed and we lose clarity. We need to be in balance in our physical, emotional, mental and spiritual lives to maintain clarity, or resonance. Any disturbance of that perfect balance and things start to show up, drawing our attention to some maintenance or corrective action that is required. It is our free will to choose to listen, or not.

Reiki is a wonderful practice where universal healing energy from Upstairs is offered to the energy field and is transmuted to whatever is needed by the body. In my experience it is not directed energy, but rather an inpouring of healing to flood the body and be picked up by whatever needs it the most. This may not be the experience of others, but it certainly was my experience. I still say Reiki remains one of my favourite therapies when I feel that I just need to be ironed out and smoothed over.

I have never come to understand anything more about my problems or needs after a Reiki session, ergo it does not inform, but my goodness does it leave me feeling so much better. My only reservation here, is that if I do not understand how I have healed, how can I prevent myself from falling back into the behaviour or situation that caused the distress in the first place. Knowledge is power and for a lasting result one needs to understand the dynamics at play. Otherwise you have just handed your healing over to someone else and have completely disempowered yourself. To make lasting, permanent change, you need to own your own healing and do your own work.

Chakras

There are many different chakra systems throughout the body, in the hands, the feet and the head. I am only going to talk about the seven main chakras. There are many books available on the subject, but for my purposes an overview is sufficient. I have learned everything I needed to know through accessing these main seven. The others are useful especially if you are working with a client who doesn't want to be touched or who is injured in some way. I'm giving you the cliff notes version as is my style. I will overlay parts of my story in the appropriate places to demonstrate the personalities of each chakra. A chakra is a series of vortices that spin either drawing energy into the body or pushing it out. Each chakra has a certain number of vortices and the more vortices, the faster the spin, or the higher the frequency.

The base chakra

The base chakra or root chakra is situated, as one might expect from the name, just below the base of the spine. It is traditionally associated with the colour red (sometimes black) and is the slowest spinning chakra with only four vortices. This chakra holds the energy and information dealing with your security, body awareness, survival, will to live, need to belong to a group or tribe, and your own connectedness to the here and now. When one is fully functional in this chakra one is referred to as grounded.

Imagine if you will, a root growing from your tailbone down into the Earth and anchoring you here in this lifetime, holding you secure. If any of these aspects are threatened as was the case when I was a child, you become ungrounded. I had a mentally ill mother who blamed me for everything that was wrong in her life and she tore my self-worth to shreds at every opportunity. I was taught to become invisible just to be acceptable to her. Because I withdrew to protect myself, I struggled to fit in with the community (a loner at school with no friends). I couldn't take part in school activities and so I was largely without community.

I became so adept at hiding in plain sight that I lost the ability to be authentically me, and this led to me adopting a series of masks throughout my life just to feel acceptable to others. I have frequently throughout my struggles with my health, lost the will to live. I actually could not bring myself to dress in the colour red until I was past the age of thirty-five. The colour made me so uncomfortable that I became irritable and combative when I wore it.

Once I understood more about chakras, I trained myself to embrace the colour red. It really does suit me. Distortions or imbalance in this chakra would explain rootless drifters, flitting from one place to another, never setting down roots, never claiming their place in the world; or the opposite distortion being the stick in the mud, who goes nowhere and does nothing, for whom life is just drudgery. Issues of physical wounding affect this chakra.

The sacral chakra

Moving up the body, the sacral chakra is positioned between the pubic bone and the navel. It is typically represented by the colour orange. It has six vortices and therefore spins faster and at a slightly higher vibration than the base. This chakra holds the energy pertaining to your personal power, issues of pleasure and creativity, vitality and sexuality. It is the fire in your belly, or your tepid response to life. Try making a bold I am statement with a blocked or distorted sacral chakra, you simply cannot do it.

For others who have the opposite distortion, they are all about the great I am, they are often the life and soul of the party, the inappropriately loud and overzealous. Also, this is where you look when your get up and go feels like it has got up and gone as mine had for most of my life. It makes perfect sense that I had great distortions in these areas. I was always playing a role that someone else determined for me, I had learned that being me was dangerous and undesirable.

The years I spent singing in church and dancing in the theatre, were my soul's way of trying to light the fire in my belly, to drive me to discover my sense of self. So great was my wounding however, that it didn't work and it took many more years before I finally found my way. Issues with your connection to your Higher Self will affect this chakra. This chakra can be read on the back and the front of the body. The front is where issues of quality and personal power sit – what is the quality of your life, do you experience pleasure and vitality and feel good about yourself. The back is where issues of quantity and abundance are to be found. Do you have enough creativity in your life, or opportunities to explore your sexuality, enough vitality to get through the day?

The solar plexus chakra

The next chakra sits above your navel in the region of your liver. It has ten vortices and spins faster and at an even higher frequency than the sacral. It is typically expressed by the colour yellow. This chakra governs issues of inter-personal power, how you relate to people and how you present yourself to the world. This chakra can also be read on the back and front of the body.

The front will tell you about your attitudes to, and responsibility for your own health, financial, social, mental, emotional, spiritual and physical needs. The back will give you your ethics, emotional issues related to responsibility, self-esteem, fear of rejection and oversensitivity to criticism. This chakra in my life was pretty much destroyed. I was determined to do everything on my own and I simply could not. When I reached out to others for help, they could not. I was rejected from the moment I was born and had no faith in the people who were supposed to protect me. I struggled with being responsible for myself and went for long periods allowing myself to suffer. This is where your emotional wounding sits.

The heart chakra

This chakra sits, as you would expect, over your heart and with twelve vortices it has the highest vibration of all the lower four chakras. The heart is represented by the colour green and deals with issues of love. Reading this chakra on the front of the body will give you an insight into your ability to give love, your connection to another person, your unconditional love and affection, friendship, compassion, empathy and loyalty.

By reading the back of the heart chakra you can find out more about your ability to let yourself be loved, your ego, your self-worth and your ability to self-love. It is abundantly clear from the stories I have shared that the back of my heart was completely closed off. I was in no way prepared to allow myself to be loved. I was all give and no take. I was taught that I was unworthy and unwanted and love was not for me. My major relationships in life had all been tainted by my not being good enough and I had absolute trust issues. However, on the front of the heart I was all give. I loved fiercely and often inappropriately, all the while giving off mixed signals and hiding my own needs for fear of being hurt. Issues of inner mothering are found in this chakra. Mothering isn't necessarily how your mother treated you, it is more about how you were nurtured, encouraged, soothed, allowed to develop either by others, or by yourself.

The throat chakra

Positioned over the throat, with sixteen vortices, this chakra spins faster than the lower four and is usually represented by a light turquoise blue. This chakra holds the information about how you express yourself to the world and the masks you wear. People with imbalances of the throat chakra are often those that whisper softly when they speak, afraid of speaking out, or they are excessively loud, drowning you out to keep you at bay. The front of this chakra holds the information pertaining to your responsibility for meeting your own needs, and acceptance of the challenge to be true to yourself.

The back of the chakra talks more about your connection to the bigger picture and your attitude towards Spirit (Upstairs). Issues of inner fathering affect this chakra. Again, this isn't about how your father treated you, but it is about how you were protected, promoted, held accountable. I rarely, if ever spoke my truth, not because I consciously decided to withhold myself, I wasn't aware until I started to unpack my Pandora's box, how I truly felt and how I was behaving. I wasn't aware that I had a furiously angry inner child with a potty mouth to match. I was largely unaware of how I felt because I had never been made to feel important enough to have an opinion. Yes, I played many roles in life, but I hid so much of myself as well. I was way past middle age before I allowed myself to believe there was a God who was even aware of my existence.

The brow chakra

Positioned mid forehead between the eyebrows, this chakra has ninety-six vortices and operates at a very high frequency. A beautiful indigo blue in colour this chakra is where all aspects of your intuition, soul knowledge, learning and wisdom are stored. On the front, you will find issues pertaining to development and trust of your intuition, and the allowing of soul knowledge to be remembered.

On the back you will find information relating to your ability to manifest and bring ideas into being by practical application of skills. Often people with imbalances here are all about the ideas and theories, or they hide out in academia gathering knowledge. They could also be those who deny themselves learning and never implement anything they think about. They are all pie in the sky and they don't take any risks. Or they could become the big ideas people of the world and live in their heads never connecting with reality.

In this chakra you will find your adult perspectives about your childhood experiences. I instinctively knew there was so much more to me than had been allowed. I learned and I experimented. I tried so many new things and I did develop my intuition rather well. However, I lacked the courage of my convictions and I allowed others to break my trust in my own capabilities. I took an incredibly long time to delve into those childhood issue to attempt to resolve them.

The crown chakra

This chakra is positioned right above the top of the head. It is expressed with a violet white colour and with almost one thousand vortices the frequency is exceptionally high. This is the closest we get to the frequency of a soul in Spirit or Upstairs. This chakra is the spiritual doorway though which you connect to, and integrate with, your whole soul. It is your connection to all that is. This chakra holds the key to unblocking your life. Having denied the existence of God/Spirit for so many years, I was clearly very blocked. I cut myself off from the very source of all that I needed to sort out my life.

I pause here a moment and think of all the wonderful people I worked with in the rehab centre, many of whom were desperately seeking their spiritual selves in the bottom of a bottle of spirits. My utter unworthiness that was ingrained in me from the moment I was born and was reinforced throughout my childhood into adulthood, made it impossible for me to accept that I had any part in the greatness that was the Kingdom of Heaven.

There is so much information available to us if we just go within and look. Ask for guidance from energy healers or practice the art of meditation and learn to read your own body. Your physical body will often mirror the state of your chakras and dis-ease and illness will show up in areas of your body that give you the clues where to look.

Resonance

Every object, including the human body resonates at an optimal frequency. Stressors can cause the body to resonate out of harmony, such as the ice when stressed by heat loses its resonance and transforms to water and so on. This disharmony can lead to dis-ease. A body humming along well fed and watered, exercised, with healthy emotions from being sufficiently loved and all needs met, will operate in a state of resonance. A body under stress will lose resonance and could become a candidate for illness.

It is well documented in the field of vibrational medicine that disharmony shows up in the energy field long before it shows up in your body. Think if you will of the etheric bodies mentioned earlier. Something is stressing your being and there is an imbalance, this could be either known or unknown to you. The resulting disharmony triggers a signal to your spiritual etheric body. If you are not tuned into your spiritual needs, or you have not learned to listen to your intuition, you may miss the message.

Remember also that this etheric operates at a very high vibrational frequency and it takes practice to hear what it is telling you. Next the message comes through at a slower frequency and you might at this stage get an inkling that something isn't quite right. Your mental etheric body has registered a slight unease with you, but you still brush it aside and carry on with your busy life.

Next the signal gets slowed right down and triggers your emotional etheric body. Here you start to feel out of sorts and maybe get a bit irritable or feel irrationally sensitive. You are having an emotional reaction to the feeling of discomfort. Still you brush it aside, put in an extra hour at the gym to boost your energy and the message remains unheard.

Next it pings in your physical etheric body and it shows up as twinges, or feelings of lack, or maybe even a headache. Still you don't pay attention and so finally in a desperate attempt to get your attention, your actual body goes into a state of dis-ease. Corrective measures have not been taken and so physical symptoms show up that may finally force you to stop and pay attention. A migraine headache, a cold, a sprained ankle and any other symptom up to and including cancer.

These are generally all signs that there is a disharmony in your life and that something is out of balance. Nature craves resonance and everything in your body will fight to regain that state of harmony, but if you do not heed the warning signs and address the cause of the problem, the body will go on strike. To continue in a state of disharmony could cause irreparable damage and so the body attempts to make you listen. It is like a testy toddler hanging onto your leg going, "Mom, Mom, Mom, Mommy, Ma, Mama, MOTHER!!!" The sooner you learn to listen, the more likely you are to get back into a state of resonance.

There are many ways to repair damage to the human body. One can use the senses,

- hearing (listen to some music),
- smell (go into the mountains with the fresh air, woody aromas and earthiness),
- taste (make sure you are eating loads of beautiful fresh fruit and vegetables),
- sight (go down to the shore and take in the view across the bay, or go to an art exhibition) and
- touch (get a massage or have a Reiki treatment).

This will work for minor transgressions and imbalances. However, if your distress and disharmony is caused by poor lifestyle choices or latent unresolved trauma, stronger corrective actions may be needed. Once illness has set in, you may need to see health practitioners and there are so many disciplines to choose from. Here are some that I have tried.

For touch therapy you might look at, physiotherapy, Reiki, massage, hot stones, aromatherapy, or reflexology.

For natural medicines you could try flower remedies, herbal medicines or homeopathy.

For breathing or relaxation there is meditation, breath work, dancing, sports, or hypnosis.

Finally there are many areas of energy healing including, but not limited to, chiropractic, shiatsu, crystal therapy, aura soma colour therapy and spiritual healing.

There is also frequency medicine including Rife, Scio, Biofeedback; and other alternative diagnostic methods such as Iridology and Live blood analysis or kinesiology; plus for your emotional and mental well-being you might try talk therapy, hypnotherapy or life coaching. No one can say I didn't try. Of course, there is also allopathic medicine and the good old medical profession. I hope you have better luck with them than I did.

Unfortunately, sometimes the disharmony in our bodies defies explanation and despite visiting half the health care professionals in town as well as most of the alternative guys, you simply cannot arrive at a diagnosis which means no action plan and no corrective actions are being taken. Your state of disharmony intensifies and your whole system collapses.

This is where I find the psychics, the mediums and the Inner Tuition people incredibly helpful. Because they are working within the energy field, they are able to pick up the information stored there and can often point you in the right direction. It's up to you of course, to do the work and affect your own healing, but it is nice when you get a road map. By using what I'd learned from all my teachers and finally through Inner Tuition, I found the answers I was looking for, inside of myself. They had been there all along, I simply hadn't been in a position to listen or see.

I remember visiting a psychic once shortly before the Dubai trip and the retrenchment drama. My health was terrible, I was struggling so hard. I was losing my words and I couldn't stay awake. My breathing was erratic and my body hurt. Everything just felt too hard. My family history included heart disease and cancer and I was well aware that as an overweight, underactive woman in her fifties I was a sitting duck waiting for trouble.

When I started experiencing chest pains and excessive sweating, I started to panic a bit. My GP at the time had said she couldn't find anything wrong. So once again I resorted to the world of weird shit for answers. When I arrived at the psychic's house, she came to the gate, took one look at me and said, "I can't work with you, go away."

I was stunned. I was also desperate and wasn't about to take no for an answer. I heard myself telling her to go inside and pull herself together and I would wait in the lounge until she was ready to do my reading. Truly, where do these words come from sometimes? She had her turn to be stunned then, but she showed me through to her lounge. She did indeed take a ten-minute hiatus before she joined me and asked gruffly, "So what do you want?" Nice!

All I wanted to know, through her, from my Spirit Guides, was did I still have time to turn this all around? In the end we had a wonderful reading and it was very informative. I apparently did have time provided I began immediately to take better care of myself. It's not that I haven't been trying to for years, but seriously where does a girl have to go to get some bloody support and help? I asked her why she hadn't wanted to work with me and she told me she hadn't ever come across a person with an aura so completely shattered into a million pieces and she had been afraid she would be the one to finally cause a total disintegration. I have skated very close to the line on many occasions.

I consulted a cardiologist for a stress ECG and check-up. I ended up having a full-blown asthma attack on the treadmill. His response was that I should find a lung guy, he only did hearts and by the way mine was just fine as far as he could tell. If I wasn't prepared to run any faster, he really couldn't be absolutely sure, but he was sufficiently satisfied that I was okay.

Next stop lung doctor who diagnosed chronic obstructive pulmonary disease. He told me to get off the cortisone once and for all and to use preventative inhalers instead. He also said I was not to even consider flying to Dubai, I was far too sick. I figured, what the hell did he know? I only had asthma during springtime and the rest of the year I was fine, so how could I have COPD. I flew and I'm so glad I did.

Chapter 36

The clearing of Pandora's box

Drawing from my corporate days, there are certain models that I find highly informative and when overlaid with the energy work are incredibly enlightening. There is good old Maslow's Hierarchy of Needs. This is a motivational theory in psychology comprising a five-tier model of human needs, often depicted as hierarchical levels within a pyramid. Needs lower down in the hierarchy must be satisfied before individuals can attend to needs higher up. From the bottom of the hierarchy upwards, the needs are physiological, safety, love and belonging, esteem and self-actualization.

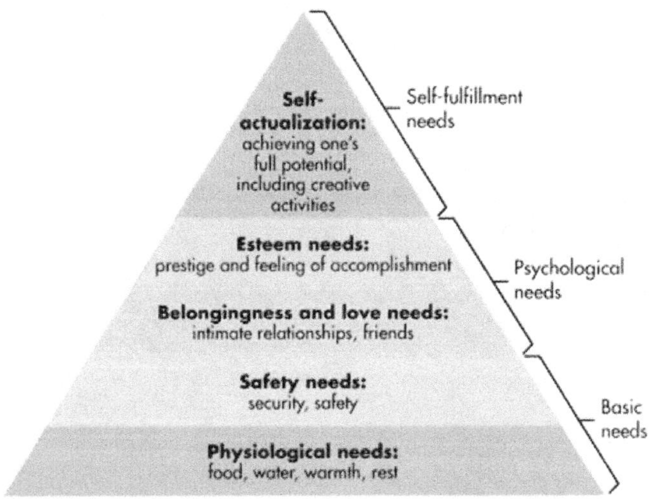

In my case I always had my physiological needs met, but that was where it ended. I have never felt completely safe or secure and therefore everything else above that was built on shaky ground. That is why when I was berated by my friend for daring to do energy work at the rehab centre without a degree in psychology, I wasn't secure enough to stand my ground and I crumbled. I never fully trusted the friendships and relationships in my life and I learned that that was because the safety and security issues didn't allow me to. This in turn led to a lack of self-esteem. My accomplishments were not being driven by my needs, rather by the needs of others I sought to gain approval from. Of course, self-actualisation and reaching that dreaded potential just wasn't in the cards for me at all since I had no solid grounding beneath me.

If you look at the bottom two tiers physiological and safety needs, you will notice that they coincide with the characteristics governed by the base chakra; belonging and love needs are the jurisdiction of the heart chakra; and the esteem and self-actualisation dovetail nicely into the crown chakra. I was beginning to see where I needed to look. Inner Tuition teaches the importance of the Base, Heart, Crown triad. Think of my simple philosophy, I am a spiritual being (Crown – connected to all that is), having a human experience (Base – living here on planet Earth), through the medium of love (Heart – expressing love and allowing yourself to receive love, or not).

Those are absolutes in my mind and they make up the framework for the human experience. Interestingly the other chakras, sacral – how you define yourself and how much energy you put into your life; solar plexus – how you emote and deal with your feelings and interpersonal relationships; throat – whether you speak your truth or throttle yourself and hide behind your masks; and brow – whether you learn, acquire knowledge, allow and listen to your intuition and apply what you know to manifest your desired reality; well those are all choices you make. We talk about those four as being part of a washing machine cycle. We can tumble around in those four chakras making self-limiting choices, holding ourselves back, chopping and changing our minds, until we are completely washed out. However, when they are balanced against the solid framework of the Base, Heart, Crown, they can be calmed down and one can find one's true rhythm in life. All it takes is the courage to look inward and the desire to make a change.

The next model I love is Johari's Window (diagram on next page). This is a construct that helps people better understand their relationship with themselves and others. It was created by psychologists Joseph Luft and Harrington Ingham in 1955 and is used primarily in self-help groups and corporate settings as a heuristic exercise.

The Johari Window

1 Open Known to self and to others	2 Blind Not known to self but known to others
3 Hidden Known to self but not to others	4 Unknown Not known to self or others

The Open area is also called the Arena. This is the space we play in where we willingly expose ourselves to others. The Blind spot holds those things about us that we are unaware of, but that are seen by others. This would be where the wretched potential might fit in. The Hidden area is also known as the Façade, this is the space where we hide aspects of ourselves from others. This can be a self-protective mechanism or it can be manipulative.

The Unknown is that which is still to be discovered by anyone. This is the playground of the chakras. If you want to blow your Johari Window wide open, examine the information stored in your chakras. I think I found out so much about myself when I finally did the work, that I shot a catapult right through my window and smashed it to smithereens. Writing this book is the equivalent of throwing my window wide open and allowing anyone who cares to look a right eyeful. It's a little scary (learned pattern of behaviour still trying to keep a grip on me), and it is also incredibly liberating. It is a huge relief to finally be free to be me.

The last model I really resonate with is from Transactional Analysis called the Parent Adult Child Model. Transactional analysis is a psychoanalytic theory and method of therapy based on the idea that one's behaviour and social relationships reflect an interchange between parental (critical and nurturing), adult (rational), and childlike (adaptive and free) aspects of personality established early in life. It is possible to adjust your behaviour by being aware of the state of your ego.

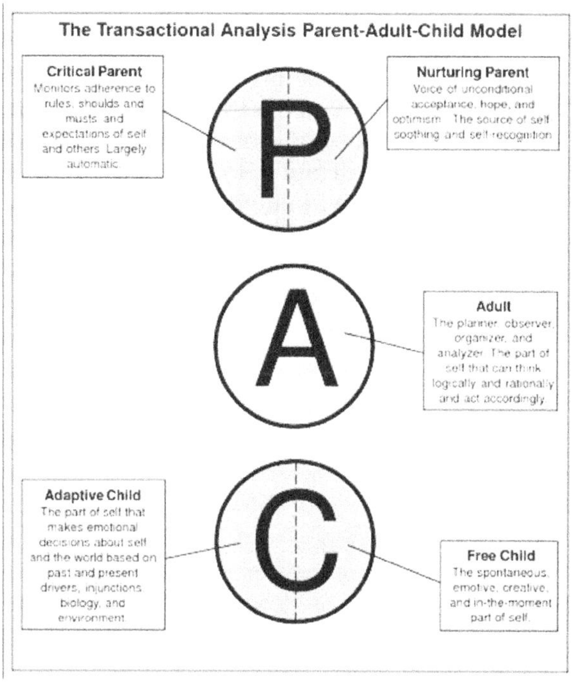

Using this model, I was able to examine my behaviours and see which role I was playing in each situation I was trying to deal with. I found it almost impossible to be in an adult state of mind until I had revisited every nasty, sticky piece of my history and made my peace with it. I had a lot of self-reclamation to do before I could become a balanced adult. The goal with each interpersonal transaction is that both parties are okay with the exchange. I had so much to learn.

When Mother came at me in her full-blown critical parent ego state as dictated by *them,* I morphed into my adaptive child. I made fear-based choices and decisions to hide myself in order to avoid her censure. I had learned from previous experience and my Father's example, that the path of least resistance led to the least amount of pain and suffering. I struggled to relate to other children who were free spirited and spontaneous. Nothing in me could relate to their seemingly dangerous behaviour because I hadn't experienced nurturing on any level that was meaningful to me. I had no belief that things would be ok and I wasn't safe enough to feel free.

In a bid to understand myself better, I first had to accept that there may be reasons I didn't fully grasp, that were governing my actions. I also had to accept that just because something triggered a response in me, didn't mean I had to act on it. I also needed to figure out what it was that made me feel worthwhile and valuable as a person. What it was that made it so hard for me to accept myself as I was and to be kind to myself. If I could learn to choose my response, I could influence a situation instead of becoming a victim to it. I also had to accept that I had a natural born right to choose joy, health and happiness, instead of stress, fear and pain. Inner Tuition taught me that self-love and self-appreciation come from self-knowledge. It was time to go down the rabbit hole.

Chapter 37

A defining moment

It took me two years of almost constant sobbing, hand wringing and utter anguish before I stopped thrashing around and finally made peace with myself. Looking back, I realised I had stumbled blindly through my childhood; spent my twenties focussed on everyone and everything else to the total exclusion of what I needed; ached my way through my thirties in total denial; wheezed my way through my forties; and I was limping my way through my fifties. I had been reduced to a shell of myself as ability after ability was stripped from my life; as symptom after symptom threatened to overwhelm me.

I had lost my ability to work. My child rearing days were done. I could no longer be gainfully employed. I had lost my independence and my home, the two things that represented my ability to take care of myself. I had lost so many friends and great acquaintances. Relationships take work and when you aren't in a position to show up, let alone reciprocate, you become quickly forgettable. I had no animals in my life except for ex-Husband's cat who hated me on sight and refused to be in the same room as me.

I felt cut off from everything in life that represented joy to me, singing, dancing, riding, travelling, time with friends. All I had left was the weird shit and even that was challenging because of my physical limitations. I had pulled through this far on sheer bloody mindedness, coupled with a stubborn refusal to lie down and die, although I had flirted with that option on more occasions than could be considered healthy. I used my seething anger and righteous indignation at the unfairness of it all to fan the flames in me that were flickering ever lower and lower.

My final flirtation with dying happened during an Inner Tuition class. Once again, I was BOB (body on bed) and the facilitator was demonstrating inner child work. She loved using me as BOB because I was so deliciously messed up it was easy to demonstrate the information to the students. Different student body, same rabbit hole/pitfall/gaping chasm.

I had been going through a very rough patch, this was at the stage where I had the twisted gut going on (it hadn't been revealed to me yet). I was so weak and in so much pain I could barely put one foot in front of the other. My belly was blown up like a blimp and I felt so uncomfortable. I felt as though my batteries had been removed. The only thing I registered was pain. I was exhausted and desperate and I couldn't see any way forward. I had taken care of myself by going to a health farm, I had embraced veganism which had just made me more ill.

No doctors had any answers for me, they all told me there was nothing wrong, or they labelled me with diagnoses that were complete rubbish. I was sick and tired and I'd had enough of struggling. What was I even struggling for? One of the students said to me, "What's wrong, you have no colour today. Normally you are a swirl of red and yellow and orange, but today you are all grey." That was a pretty accurate description of how I felt, bleak and grey and colourless.

I clambered up onto the bed and they began by checking the spins on my chakras. There was absolutely no movement anywhere except at my crown chakra, and that was only the faintest flicker of movement. The students were very uncomfortable, the facilitator was delighted. This was something she could really work with; and I couldn't have cared less. She demonstrated how to use their hands to hold one chakra secure whilst sending energy up through the one below. Once a healthy spin was achieved, they moved up the body, held the next one and sent energy up to the one previously held, and so on and so on.

I disconnected from the entire process. I was lying there with my eyes closed and I began to drift away. My breathing became more and more shallow until I was barely drawing breath at all. I felt myself dissociate from the activity and stand up out of my body. I saw myself lying on the bed surrounded by students, and I started to walk away down a long white passage. It looked a little like a hospital corridor, only cleaner and lighter.

I saw something in the distance and I walked towards it. There was a man in a white robe sitting at a table. He stood up and came towards me. He placed his hands on my shoulders and it was the most incredibly comforting feeling I have ever experienced. He looked into my eyes and said, "You need to go back, it isn't time yet. You have things to do." It was like the headmaster had said all those years ago, "This must be a mistake, go back to class." The next thing I knew, I was back on the bed with the facilitator commanding me to breathe. The students had given up trying to kick start my recalcitrant chakras and had asked the facilitator to step in.

She realised something very significant was going on for me and she held the energy. By this I mean she became a conduit for Universal energy and connected me to Spirit; plugging me into source as it were. By doing this she allowed my Spirit Guides to work with me. Remember, they are silent partners and may only intervene if asked to do so. She was asking on my behalf. My Higher Self naturally knew this wasn't my time to leave and so, by facilitating that connection I had been able to meet with someone from my Upstairs team. I'm not sure who it was, for now it isn't important, but in that one defining moment, I was firmly placed back on track and I returned to my body.

Does this mean she healed me? No. Does this mean that someone can change your karma? No. She simply facilitated an event whereby I was temporarily reconnected with my source energy, that part of me that lives in Spirit that has all the answers; who knows why I am here and what I need to accomplish; who has the ruddy project plan for my life, complete with contingencies. I had absolute free will in that transaction. I could have staged a stubborn sit in in that tunnel, possibly arranged a stroke that would have left me stuck there until my time on Earth ran out.

I could simply have refused to come back. I could have staged a crisis that would have allowed me to short circuit this lifetime. I could have kept on walking and I could have crossed over back into Spirit. It was my choice entirely to come back to my shitty, horrid life. You'll notice that I wasn't told what it was I needed to come back to do, simply that I had business to attend to. That spoke to everything in me. I was the Service to the School recipient, I was always in service to someone, some cause, something else. That simple connection with the energy of pure love, was enough to reawaken my desire to live and relit my pilot light, the fire in my belly, my sacral chakra that holds the energy of the I am statement.

I had been granted a miniscule insight into what is waiting for us back in Spirit. If that small touch on my shoulder is anything to go by, well it's going to be wonderful indeed. I understand why my Dad and my sister's partner had given me such glowing and wonderful feedback. They are existing in a state of bliss. I now realised there was nothing to fear in dying, it truly is the greatest reward at the end of a life, but since I had come so far already and someone on that side believed in my ability to deliver, I might as well get down to business and find out what it was that I was here to do.

No one in that session that day knew anything about what I had experienced. The facilitator asked me to stay behind after class. She knew something significant had gone down and she was curious. This is why we always work under guidance of Spirit and we ask for protection when doing energy work. Protection goes three ways, protection for the facilitator, protection for the client, and protection for the process. The students were protected from a traumatic experience, watching me die on the bed. The facilitator was protected from the process taking place. She was a completely hollow conduit through which the energy flowed, thus keeping her ego totally out of the process – this wasn't her business to deal with.

I was protected from myself. I was allowed to travel safely to a different dimension to obtain a little more information with which I could make an informed choice to stay or leave this life. When she had commanded me to breathe, that must have been the moment I made my decision. I had actually stopped breathing on her bed. If she had known what I was experiencing, pandemonium would have resulted. Panic would have taken over, paramedics would have been called and I would probably now be sitting on a fluffy white cloud trying to figure out how I could build a better life plan for the next incarnation so that I might actually get to master what it is I have come here to do. I have been told by more than one psychic that I am on my fourth lifetime with the same lesson. There is no way I want to do this again, so I am thrilled that it all worked out the way it did. I love this weird shit.

Even with everything I know and everything I have experienced I still have moments when my indoctrinations as a human give me pause. I get to choose whether to stay this path or not. Free will can be a real bugger! I remember when I explained the world of energy to the youngsters in the rehab, they would say to me, "What happens if you're wrong?" and I used to hear myself say, "What happens if I'm right?" Now, at this point in my life I finally understand what I was teaching those gorgeous lost souls, I was teaching them to dare to question for themselves what was right or wrong. I was teaching them to look inside for the answers. I was teaching them that they were more beautiful and powerful than they could ever know or accept and I was offering them the permission they felt they needed to start exploring that possibility.

Chapter 38

Time to take a good long look

It had all started that day at the hairy therapist where, under hypnosis, I had experienced my birth. Almost two decades later I decided it might be time to fully explore that situation. I'd had the most incredible experience that had changed my life and challenged everything I knew. Yet I hadn't received any support or instructions for how to process that information. In absolute honesty, I have to own the fact that the reason for that huge transgression of trust, sits fairly and squarely with me. The weirdness of the circumstances and the utter shittiness of what I had experienced was so overwhelming, I ran, hard and fast in the opposite direction. It was exactly the same with the meditation workshop where I had been personally greeted by Spirit through a pretty blonde woman speaking in a Jamaican man's voice. I got scared and I ran away. It was such weird shit that I was terrified.

By this stage of life however, I knew enough about the weird shit to know that the hypnosis session was only the tip of the iceberg. I decided to allow myself to go back to that time and really see what was going on. Understanding that I was going back with an adult mindset, a full set of reasoning skills and the knowledge that Mother was mentally ill, I allowed myself through meditation and journey work, to explore the link between my being held (meeting my most primal need) and being fed (another base need).

I finally explored my relationship with food. I discovered that I did not find food a comfort at all. Quite the opposite in fact. I was using food as a tool to punish myself and make myself as unlovable as possible, because that was how I had felt as a new arrival, completely ignored and discounted, ergo unlovable. I was held when I was fed and so food represented a punishment to me. I wanted to leave and not live, and yet they kept on feeding me and keeping me alive. I felt so unlovable that I learned to eat to make myself invisible. I ended up attracting to myself the very censure that I had been taught to expect as the child of a mentally ill primary caretaker.

I became a self-fulfilling prophesy. If I was fat enough, no one would bother to look at me or take me seriously and I could remain invisible. I have to say here that the fact that it worked so well, makes me terribly sad. I long for a time when humanity will assess a person's worth based on the openness of their heart, rather than the size of their waistlines or their butts. I have some very dear friends who simply cannot see past my size and I am fully aware of how my value is diminished in their eyes because of their prejudice.

I firmly believe that once my body is finally functioning correctly, the weight problems will resolve. For the most part I no longer buy into others' opinions of me and I know I am not diminished by being overweight. This is an ongoing learning process though and I suspect it will continue throughout my life. I feel compelled to honesty here and I have to admit I still find that part challenging. I am, at times, very vulnerable to what I feel is the censure of others, or a lack of understanding of me perhaps.

I accept that I am the one who has been sending out mixed signals and I am the one who has changed the status of our connection. I remain optimistic though that as I learn to accept and respect myself, others will see that I am showing them how to treat me. I am setting a better example by treating myself with respect and kindness. I have decided to simply stop focussing on food as a protagonist, a culprit, or a solution in my journey and I will let the chips fall where they may with regards to my size. There are far more important things to focus on in life and I am delighted to be free of this lifelong struggle.

As an aside, I did once join an online dating site and I was contacted by a chap who was very excited to meet me. He confessed to having a fetish for overweight gals and he couldn't wait to roll around in my fleshy wonderland. Ugh! I recommended he see a therapist and took down my profile immediately. Good grief!

I was co-facilitating an Inner Tuition course and we had the most amazing group of students. We dubbed them the Whacky Wednesday Girls and my goodness but we had some experiences together. We were starting the dreaded inner child work and having explained all about the wounded child, we began a practical demonstration of how to access the inner child via the chakras. I was the designated BOB (body on bed) and the facilitator was running the session. The students went into a meditative state and tried to tune into what I was experiencing. We were looking for anything that was relevant to my state of health and we were hoping to find clues as to where I might begin unravelling my health conundrum.

The moment the facilitator connected with my inner child I was that ten-month-old baby again being tossed into my cot on my head. It was a surreal experience to be able to feel what that little baby had felt and to realise that although I had decided to stop crying as a matter of self-preservation, I was in fact, so angry, that I could have spontaneously combusted. I was able to feel that immense anger and I was stunned that such a tiny baby could have such enormous passion. I felt what I can only describe as feral.

Worse than that though was when I looked up into Mother's eyes and she snarled at me with such a venom and hatred it almost stopped my breath, "Just bloody get on with it then, I've had enough of you! I wish to Christ you had never been born!" That last part was a new revelation, but it was the tone of her voice that chilled my blood. I have only heard that degree of hatred one other time in my life and that was the day I told her that she was moving to a nursing home. She looked at me with that same hatred in her eyes and in that exact tone of voice she said, "Are you happy now? You have finally taken everything from me." Now I could finally understand that response as well.

One of the ladies had managed to tune into this delightful little episode and I was gratified to find her sitting on the couch looking like a stunned mullet after we had finished. She was felled by the extent of the pain that I had been exposed to and she had no way to process it. She could not understand how someone could harbour such hatred for their own child. Somehow this validated me enormously because I realised I wasn't imagining this or catastrophising a situation. I truly had been through a traumatic ordeal. I was entitled to my feelings.

It took me a long time to come to terms with the fact that my own Mother had hated me and had wished I had never been born. I had to balance that out with the fact of her mental illness and in time, I realised that it actually wasn't personal. It wasn't about me at all. She was battling her own demons and possibly because her symptoms started right after my traumatic birth, I became the focal point for her instability and she blamed it all on me.

She had no more control over her actions, than I had control over my emotions. She probably did regret having a baby so late in life and I'm sure having me scream my head off for ten long months day and night didn't help matters either. I spent many sessions in talk therapy going around and around this scene, but I couldn't find my way out of it, or past it. I made the decision to stop therapy and try a life coach instead. The wonderful distinction between the two in my experience is that where the therapist went back and unpacked the situation to find out why I was stuck, the coach started with where I was and helped me find a way to move forward.

I was tired of going over and over this scene, refuelling the pain and getting nowhere. It took three sessions with the coach for me to be able to put this issue down once and for all and leave it alone. My needs immediately after birth had not been met. I had made a reptilian brain decision that life wasn't worth living, kind of like stop the ride I want to get off. When I couldn't get off, I had protested loudly and with much fury until Mother reached her point of no return.

That awful moment at the beginning of my life, was finally transmuted from a three headed monster that threatened to consume me, to nothing more than a one-dimensional inert representation of my history, a cave painting as it were. It had happened yes, it was painful yes, my response to it had knocked me right off course yes, but it no longer had the power to wound me. I was finally free.

I spent some time in meditation and taking along my Higher Self for good measure, I went back to that room with my new-found peace of mind. I picked up that little baby and I sang to her and I rocked her and I soothed all the anger right out of her. I held her until she squirmed, and then I tucked her inside my heart and reclaimed that part of me that had been lost for so long. I put down my sword and I decided to stop fighting and start living. I made my peace with what had happened and I released the energy of the situation back to the Universe and replaced it with unconditional love for that tiny unloved part of me. In doing so, I freed myself from my lifelong struggle.

There are still moments when people speak to me with the energy or tone of Mother's voice that gives me sharp pause. However, for the most part I am able to be still and allow the emotion to pass and make a healthy decision about how to respond. This is also largely contingent upon me taking really good care of myself. If I overdo things and stretch myself too thin, stressing my ailing body or my limited energy, I become debilitated and can spiral down into the depths of my all too familiar despair. By employing the tools I have learned along the way and with the self-knowledge that I have gained, I am able to bring myself back into a resonant state far easier and with less effort each time.

Meditation is a most powerful tool. It allows you to access your memories and to go back and right wrongs, to rewrite your script and to give yourself what you needed most at a time in life where you became stuck. It allows you to reclaim your lost inner child. The more broken pieces of your life that you can fix and reclaim, the more complete you become, the more whole you are, the more you can become who you were meant to be all along, the greater clarity you achieve. It can be a painful and difficult journey, but it is so worth it.

I remember doing a meditation with a young woman in the rehab facility one day. She had fallen pregnant at a very young age and her parents had forced her to have an abortion. She was completely traumatised by this and the guilt that she experienced was so all consuming that she ended up taking drugs to numb her pain. Fast forward to her sitting with me in rehab unable to forgive herself for allowing her parents to force her to murder her baby.

We went into a meditative state and we found ourselves a comfortable place to sit and I invited her Higher Self to come and sit with us. Once she was comfortable and had quietened her mind, I asked for her Spirit Guides to bring in her baby. In that meditation she was able to hold her baby boy and pour out her heart to him and most importantly, she was able to ask him for forgiveness. I shall never forget that experience as it touched my heart so deeply. She was able to find the peace that she needed to come back to her life and heal herself. She had a lot of work to do still as she needed to work on forgiving her parents and herself, but she was at peace with her baby. I'm glad that she was in rehab when she went through this because she needed some very powerful support to complete this work and I doubt she could have done it on her own.

One of my favourite learnings from Inner Tuition came when we discussed listening and what a surprisingly huge skill it is. I often quote this particular reference and I find it has helped me be mindful of not overstepping other's boundaries in my earnest, if misguided, attempts to save someone else, or to try and prevent them from experiencing pain. *When you do something for someone else that they can and should be doing for themselves, you are showing them that you have no faith in their ability to take care of themselves.* Too much love can also be disempowering. I have been guilty of great disrespect in this regard and I have worked hard to teach myself to curb my inner warrior and to support and hold those I love and care about, rather than to do for them and fix them.

Anyone who tells you they can remove your demons, change your karma, or anything along those lines needs to be treated with great caution. No one can change anything for you with any lasting effect. Only you can make a significant and lasting change in your own life by understanding your triggers and your emotional responses. It is necessary to make new decisions to fulfil the underlying needs you have, and most importantly new actions that support your new way of being are essential. Therapists, friends, support groups, anyone in the caring or healing professions can help you with the process by informing you and teaching you what is possible; and most critically by holding up a mirror for you to take a long hard look at yourself and to find your own truth. The work, however, lies fairly and squarely on your shoulders to do or not as you choose.

Many therapies are comforting, but uninformative, so while they help you to feel better the result is unlikely to be long lasting. Balancing your chakras will set your body in a state of resonance, however the minute you get up off the bed and begin to agitate and tumble around in your mind again, you immediately go back into a state of imbalance. Someone once asked me what the point of a therapy was if it couldn't fix you. Well putting your body back into a resonant state affords it much needed relief. It also allows you to connect with the feeling of resonance. Some of us have gone so far out of balance that we have come to accept discomfort as our normal state and we do not know, or remember, what it feels like to be balanced. It is much easier to aim for something if you know what it is and what it feels like. If you want the results to be long lasting, then you need to do the work to support that.

I watched a fascinating TED Talk on how childhood trauma affects health across a lifetime. Quoting from the synopsis of her talk:

"Childhood trauma isn't something you just get over as you grow up. Paediatrician Nadine Burke Harris, explains that the repeated stress of abuse, neglect and parents struggling with mental health or substance abuse issues has real, tangible effects on the development of the brain. This unfolds across a lifetime, to the point where those who've experienced high levels of trauma are at a triple the risk of heart disease and lung cancer. An impassioned plea for paediatric medicine to confront the prevention and treatment of trauma head-on."

I dived into this new area. This was something I hadn't explored before. I read so many books written by children of alcoholic or drug abusing parents, describing how the trauma of their childhoods had led them down a rabbit warren of inexplicable illness and often depression. I also learned from reading books by experts in the field of child psychology, that an emotionally or physically wounded child, can often end up facing issues of:

- co-dependency,
- offender behaviours,
- narcissistic disorders,
- trust issues,

- acting in (inappropriate self-soothing behaviours such as sex, alcohol, drugs, eating problems)
- or acting out (combative behaviours, aggression, destructive tendencies, fighting),
- magical beliefs (being away with the fairies and denying reality, waiting for someone to rescue them),
- non-disciplined behaviours,
- addictive/compulsive behaviours, thought distortions, and feelings of emptiness (apathy and depression).

These are all attributable to the distortions of love experienced by a child growing up with ongoing trauma. Once again there are many books available on this subject, and I am simply giving you a cliff notes version of my takeaway understanding.

I turned to Inner Tuition to explore my world of inner wounding. I discovered that wounding continues right through one's lifetime and can have a profound effect on our clarity of thinking. I'll explain a bit more about childhood wounding in a bit. For now, here's a simple analogy that can demonstrate the effects of trauma on a life. Imagine if you will, that you are on this journey called life. You arrive on an airplane and since your means of travelling through this life is by car, you collect yours at the parking lot outside the arrivals lounge.

If you have planned an easy life you might arrive to find a coupe waiting for you, or a nice safe family vehicle. For my life I arrived and was given the keys to a monster truck. I should have known right then that this would be a rough ride. Is it any wonder then, that my first instinct was to get the hell out of Dodge? Settling into the driver's seat you strike out. Unfortunately, you have lost your road map (remember you forgot your life plan when you were being born or left it on the plane as it were), but you are game to get going anyway and start exploring this lifetime. In my case I cautiously inched forward, I had an automatic license and had been given a stick shift.

The vehicle is brand new with no dents or scratches and you can see where you are going through the crystal-clear, clean windscreen. In my case the process of being born and of not having my immediate needs met was my first trauma. At that point the blue bird of happiness that was flying overhead shat on my wind screen. If I'd had a parent worthy of the title, she might have wiped my windscreen clean and I would have proceeded unimpeded. But that was not my experience.

When Mother tossed me into my cot, head-first, a giant blue crane unleashed a massive poop that splatted across my line of vision. At every junction where something gave me pause or knocked me off balance, another dollop of poop landed. For smaller affronts, being referred to snidely as mistress of ill health, flying insects splattered onto my window. There were road signs everywhere pointing me in the right direction. Meditation classes with Jamaican voices emanating from a pretty blonde woman for example, but I couldn't see properly through all the crap on my window.

I lurched along going further and further off course. Particularly bad swerves such as hearing my child being car jacked, was the equivalent of having a tree branch shatter my wind screen. On the odd occasion I actually swerved so hard, like when I bailed on the rehab job that I went off road completely. I ended up lost in a jungle with a dented fender and a flat tyre. Crashing along through life, unable to see with any clarity where I was going, I went further and further off course, rendering my bodywork rather the worse for wear. With every limiting decision I made, or signpost that I missed, I veered left instead of going straight and another blight was added to my vehicle.

Understand that at any stage in life, one can stop and have repairs done, or simply clean the windscreen, but when you fear that the jungle you are thrashing through is infested with tigers, you become disinclined to stop. Eventually, with enough stress, even a monster truck will stall. At some junction it becomes imperative that you at the very least, clean the darned window so that you can see where you are going. Sometimes you may need to actually replace the whole windscreen to change your outlook (cataract surgery). Repairs to bodywork get done after you get back on track, which is done by taking corrective measures such as following the signs, or maybe even asking for directions.

Not everyone has this experience. It all depends on what your life's journey is about, what you are here to master. Some journeys (lifetimes) are, of necessity, tougher than others. Some people can drive through their entire lives with the odd splattered bug on their windscreens and they don't even notice. Yet others become a complete car wreck. Sometimes, if they have gone so far off course that there is no possibility of their project manager being able to pull them back on track, they might hit the eject button and leave this life earlier than planned. They can then recalibrate their life plan and try again next lifetime. Sometimes if the journey becomes unbearably hard, they might purposely drive their car into a tree, thus releasing them to go back to Spirit and recalibrate. There is no judgement about this. We are all doing the best we can with what we can see in front of us.

Time to take a good long look

Going back and rescuing my inner ten-month-old was tantamount to giving the windscreen a good wash. Sometimes your window cleaning (rescue operation) can be so successful, that other debris is cleared away at the same time. Not everything that gives you pause in life has to be dissected. Sometimes you just have to acknowledge that it is there and it gets cleared away as part of a bigger clean up. Each of these splotches and distortions in the way you see things, creates the filters through which you perceive and experience the world around you. Is it any wonder then that we struggle so to find our way and we misread signs and drive right by opportunities? We need to clean up our crap.

Chapter 39

The wounded inner child

I have read many books and sat through courses all offered by very learned folk on the subject of childhood wounding. Here's what I took away from them all once I had distilled down the details to the bare bones. I really do like things to be simplified. We are here to learn and grow as souls. We have specific lessons to master. However, we forget what those are during the process of being born. So, how are we to do the learning then? We have cleverly written into our life plan a cast of characters with roles to play. Their roles involve setting the right scene for us, or they maybe nudge us towards our lesson plan, or they don't. All of this facilitates our ability to work it out for ourselves. They create an environment conducive to our self-discovery. Simple? Well maybe it is and maybe it isn't, it all depends on the lesson in play.

If your lesson is, for example, one of academic self-actualisation it stands to reason that you will write into your plan a loving, supportive family with sufficient resources to afford you all the opportunities you need to enter the higher learning institutions; which is the absolute kick off point for all academic greatness. That would be the easy route. Or you might plan a lifetime with parents who live on the poverty line. They can't give you the physical resources you need, but they are wise enough to know that the way out of their predicament is through a good education. Perhaps they dedicate themselves to their menial lives in such a manner that it attracts the attention of a boss or benefactor and that person can afford you the opportunity to study. Or perhaps there is no benefactor available and no amount of wishing on a star is working for you, but your desire for higher learning is so great, that you apply yourself with great discipline and dedication to your studies and you are able, on your own merits, to apply for a scholarship. This is something you needed to do for yourself. Or another alternative might be that you are born into a family that holds no regard for learning. They managed just fine without it and so what makes you think you are important enough to go to a university. They block you at every turn. You may have a teacher who sees your potential, or a friend who opens doors for you, or it might only be in later life that you embrace your academic needs and you do it all on your own. It is also possible that by hook or by crook you miss all the signposts and opportunities you wrote into your life plan and you never become a self-actualised academic. Instead you live out your perfectly ordinary life in a blissful state of ignorance.

When you cross back into Spirit at the end of your beige, bland existence feeling perfectly content, but wholly unenlightened, you will be able to put together a more dynamic or pressing life plan that will help you to get to that level you are needing to master... next time around. Self-mastery is not an easy process. If it was, it wouldn't take us so many lifetimes to achieve it and this game here on Earth wouldn't be half as much fun.

So, you can clearly see that in all of these examples the goal remained the same. The characters in your cast either supplied what was required to achieve it; or they shone in their own way attracting the manifestation of what was required for you; or you accepted the challenge and fought your own way to the top; or you didn't. Either way your goal was achieved, or it wasn't, it was all down to you in the end.

Along the way those characters in your life might have been playing out their karmic learnings at the same time. It is both as complex and as simple as that. You have a need and you attract the solution, either through careful up-front planning in Spirit, or through the beneficence of others, because they saw your inherent value and worth; or through dogged effort and a refusal to accept anything less than your due; or your needs remain unmet.

I've learned through my studies that all of life's lessons can be broken up into three major category headings or karmas, being money, sex and power.

- Money karma might play itself out as wealth, poverty, acquisition to the exclusion of all else, and all other distortions of money.
- Sex would be interpersonal relationships on all levels. Parents and children, bosses and subordinates, teachers and students, cousins, marital partners, you name it, if it's about the dynamics between people, then it sits here.
- Power translates as personal power or self-worth. The mastery of one's own worth can be a tricky one and this is definitely my primary karma in this lifetime. In another lifetime I may have come through knowing I was an incredibly powerful person and I might have had to learn that with great power comes great responsibility. I'm sure you can imagine how that could go awry. Since I am apparently half-way through my fourth lifetime on the

> same lesson, it stands to reason I wrote in some pretty big stuff to make sure I got it this time around. In my life plan, I cast characters who would decimate my self-worth in order that I might discover it for myself. At times when my being was overly stressed, I may have drifted way off course. At that stage one of my contingencies would have come into play, I might have met a teacher who introduced me to my potential (that darned word), or I might have been sent a friend, a job, a horse, or a dog that facilitated some joy in my life. All fantastic opportunities for me to discover my worth that could very well have turned me around, or not, as it turned out.

So, back to the wounding of the children. Sounds awful doesn't it. Do not fear, you are not accountable for wounding your children and the same goes the other way too. Your parents are not accountable for wounding you. They were hired to play a role and they have played their role to the best of their ability.

I shouldn't have to say this, but I will say it anyway so that there can be no misunderstanding: I do not accept, advocate for, excuse, or condone, on any level whatsoever, child abuse in any guise or format. That is another matter entirely and is not what I am alluding to here at all. The wounds I refer to, happen in the mind of the child. They belong to the child and the child alone. Remember my entreaty to the youngsters in rehab that they needed to take responsibility for their own choices, well so it is in childhood as well.

The young brain at the time of initial wounding, may not have fully developed its reasoning skills or its ability to distinguish fact from feeling. Conclusions are drawn using the reptilian part of the brain that operates primarily on instinct. For example, when I was first born, I had a primitive need for comfort. No one comforted me. At that stage I could not see myself as a separate entity. I instinctively knew I was meant to be bonded with a host (mother) and I could only think about my needs.

I could not understand the rationale that the dying mother needed to be cared for. I certainly did not understand about incubators and such. In my reptilian brain, I drew the conclusion that I was separate, alone, unwanted and unloved. Feeling so alone and scared and having no clue why I was even there (remember I had forgotten the life plan during the birth process), I decided I no longer wanted to be here. I changed my mind. I wanted to go back where it was warm and safe and I was taken care of. Stop the ride, I want to get off. Of course, it doesn't work like that. I am born, I am here and now I get to play the game.

Was my decision the fault of my bleeding, dying mother? I think not! I had reflexively jumped to that conclusion in reaction to a set of circumstances that I had set up when planning my incarnation. Tricky birth situation – tick. Mother played her part perfectly – tick. She developed her mental illness and could not nurture me as I needed in life – tick. Father was so consumed with trying to keep Mother buttoned down, he couldn't validate me either – tick. Sister wasn't aware that any of this was going on and to her I was just her weird little sister who frankly irritated the crap out of her – tick.

At every junction I took on more and more wounding and I completely missed the point. No one did this to me. Everyone played their role to perfection. The right people came along offering to show me the way by holding up mirrors so that I might see my worth. I didn't get it, but that is not the fault of my cast members. No one did anything to me, they played out their roles perfectly, or imperfectly, as was needed and in response, I made every choice, every decision, every left turn, with the occasional right turn thrown in, all by myself.

This is my life and no one can live it for me. I am not a victim, I am the sum of all of my choices to date, rolled up with all of my potential. I am a whole and divine soul, living in a dense and often uncomfortable vibration. I am learning to experience all facets of my humanity so that I might achieve enlightenment and become at one with the light. Look at that again overlaid with information regarding chakras: My life (base chakra) is the sum of my choices, in response to distortions of love (heart chakra), with all of my potential (crown chakra). A perfect base, heart, crown triad. A functional framework for the human experience.

Alrighty then, with all of that being said, let's look at these wonderful initial wounds that are so often the springboards into our life's learning. I think that if you again, break it all down to its most simple components, there are four major wounds that take place in childhood. That initial wounding that shoves you off course, facilitating your finding your way back to your life plan. Remember if energy isn't stressed it cannot transform to a different state. We live in this dense vibrational frequency and our task is to get back to our full vibrational light form as a soul. Often, much pressure must be applied to facilitate that. The four initial wounds in my opinion are as follows:

- Abilities – we feel that we should be better at some skill or competence, be it academics, sport, parenting, caring… you choose.
- Physicality – we are only lovable and acceptable if we are a certain physical type, taller, thinner, robust, delicate, less hairy… again insert your wound here.

- Identity – in order to be acceptable, we must (or must not be), male / female, black / white, Republican / Democrat, introvert / extravert, gay / straight. You name it, it all sits here.
- Connection – we can only be loved if we are, smart, successful, compliant, willing, malleable, loud, gentle… the manner in which we connect with others becomes a condition for us being acceptable or lovable… insert your condition here.

All of these wounds can be played out in the positive or negative sense.

A wounding of *abilities* might play itself out as follows: A child is born to a sporting family. Let's make them British well to do folk. They have a large estate with hounds and horses and they proudly host the annual fox hunting gala event each season. Think Downton Abbey and you are in the right vicinity. They are well set in their ways and their life works really well for them. As babies, the children are briskly walked in the bracing fresh air by nannies. As soon as they are old enough to stand, they are balanced on the back of fat little ponies.

All goes well until they fall off the pony and hurt themselves. Shocked and horrified they start to wail, expressing themselves most furiously to let everyone know they do not really like the ponies. They would really rather be playing with their dolls in the comfort of their warm nursery. Mummy and Daddy rush along and briskly brush them off, telling them not to be so silly. Riding is wonderful and how will they ever join the hunt if they keep falling off. Do stop that crying, there's nothing to cry about. They plonk them back on the pony and watch with pride as their child *bucks up* and embraces their fate.

They feel great pride as their child gallantly trots on, having been taught exactly how they need to be in order to fit in with their parent's version of what their life should and therefore will be like. They have parented their children to the best of their ability in line with what they know. The child's little brain with no ability to reason properly might decide two things; in order to be acceptable, they need to ride, and / or they are not allowed to have their own feelings. If they are hurt, they mustn't cry. They decide that in order to be loved, they have to become what their parents expect of them and so they determine to suppress themselves, complete with all their authentic feelings and they learn to ride.

A wound of *physicality* may play out in this way: "I cannot love you little one, because you are not pretty enough," said no parent ever. However, when the little one in question sees how much everyone admires their new sibling and praises them for their beauty and their lovely features, a little reptilian brain may decide, "In order to be loved and accepted by my family, I need to be beautiful." The parent's admiration and positive reinforcement of the one child, becomes the wounding of the other.

Wholly unintentional and an absurd charge to levy against the parents. You can see the people with this type of wounding often hiding beneath their carefully painted (sometimes surgically remodelled) faces, in their well-constructed and beautifully appointed homes, all surrounded by perfect exteriors. Or they might become the antithesis of what they believe is needed to become lovable, they refuse to groom or dress as expected, they are rebellious about where they live and what they surround themselves with.

They decide to challenge what they see as your restrictions to their right to be loved in order to see if you can still love them, even as they dare to be different. These rebellious souls might actually find out that their worth has nothing to do with what their reptilian brain decided for them, or they might live out a life denying themselves access to being loved. Every soul has a different experience.

Wounds of *identity* happen all the time in every walk of life. So much of the racial tension in the world stems from this particular initial wounding. You have too much privilege, or not enough. Your gender is not clearly definable, you are therefore unacceptable. Political parties sit on opposite sides of the arena pelting one another with contempt.

I once knew a married couple with opposing political views. Each felt unable to love the other unless they capitulated to their way of thinking and they ended up divorced. Society has this heinous collective term: minorities. In my opinion, everything about that word is dripping with disdain, clearly positioning the members of such groups as somehow being less than, or inferior, for having the sheer temerity to be different.

In a society largely struggling with fear, that which is not in (known, understood, same), must be kept out (corralled, limited and suppressed), a parent will raise their child according to the dictates of their particular belief system and moral code, using their ethnic, religious and community rules for guidelines and structure. A child for whom this does not resonate, may well end up wounded, deciding that they are unlovable. They find no way within the structure of their upbringing, to explore their potential, or to express themselves authentically. They are taught to be compliant to the wishes and needs of their caretakers or teachers to be acceptable. They might decide that their right to be loved is conditional upon them fitting in, being someone or something, they inherently know they are not. This is a pretty uncomfortable way of living. These people either supress themselves completely and remain a part of their silent minorities, or they might become a voice for change. There are so many different permutations of those two choices, but I think the point of the wounding is clear enough.

A wounding in the area of *connection* is a tough one to work with. Imagine being a softly spoken, gentle soul and being born to a loud, gregarious family. Family gatherings are crowded, loud, over the top celebrations of life, liberty and justice. Music is played and people dance around singing and shouting, alcohol flows freely and the revelry knows no limits. Everything in the way you connect to others is decried as wrong by your parents.

You learn that in order to be acceptable and loved, you need to be something other than your authentic self. The young man I met working at the rehab centre may well have had this as his initial wounding. He was a gentle boy with the soul of a poet. He was here to lead a peaceful existence. His father was the polar opposite of him. The father made it clear how he expected the boy to behave and comport himself in order to be acceptable, whilst his mother tried to make space for him to develop his sensitivity. This only put him right in the firing line for bully dad. This young man ended up with two opposing wounds and it is no wonder he tried to escape into the temporary oblivion of the drug world. His choice of avoidance almost cost him his life. He was so far off track with his life plan, that he reached an escape hatch clause (one of his contingencies). I do hope he managed to find his way back.

Chapter 40

Mask wearing

In each of the scenarios above we have a set of parents doing their best to raise their child using everything they have at their disposal. Remember that the parents are souls too and they are probably still harbouring their own initial wounds. Their perceptions of all that is may well be as distorted, if not more distorted, than yours. Can you see how complex it can become, or alternatively, how deliciously simple it is to unscramble?

- Step one: admit to yourself that you are not comfortable with your way of being and that it no longer serves you
- Step two: decide to stop pretending to be something or someone you are not
- Step three: examine your life and identify your wounding
- Step four: look behind your mask and discover your true self
- Step five: acknowledge that you are where you are, through your own free will regardless of your circumstances
- Step six: rebrand yourself in authenticity

Well at this point I am fully aware that what I have just said may have pissed off many people reading this book. That is excellent! Firstly, it means people are reading my book – yay! It also means that I have stirred something in you that needed a twirl. Some of you, who are still living inauthentic lives may have felt a yearning to change, which is wonderful! Others may already be in the process of learning to embrace their authentic selves, but they are nowhere near ready to admit that it is anything other than a challenging, difficult process. I am so incredibly happy for you, hang in there it does get better. Yet others, who are still living lives determined by those initial wounds, may have felt anger. How dare I say it is a simple fix when I have no idea how dreadful their existence is, or how they have been forced into their circumstances by things beyond their control. That too is wonderful. If this gets you thinking about those things outside of your control, then it is possible that something I have explained in the previous pages, may give you pause to see with a slightly altered perspective, the part that you played in it all. That is thrilling!

There may also be others who decide that I am talking utter rubbish, everything I say is outside of their experience, what they have been taught, or what is deemed acceptable within the confines of their religious teachings. They may well toss the book into the bin and get on with living their satisfying, safe, ordinary lives. I am very happy for you too. It was lovely meeting you up to this point. Perhaps in the future something that you read here will ping on your radar if the right circumstances present; and if not, then that is exactly as it should be, for you.

Nothing in life is really a problem, until it becomes a real problem for you; until it becomes unsustainable as a way of living and the need for change rears its head and can no longer be denied. Since the only way to self-mastery is through introspection and learning, I couldn't be happier for you all. Seek and you shall find! I have lived over five and a half decades either unaware, or in denial of the fact that I have had complete responsibility for my own life and my experience of it all along.

This is my play, my life plan that I chose to be here to engage with. I have had the choice at every shitty junction, to decide how to respond. Where I am now, is down to every choice I ever made. It really doesn't matter what might have happened to me, or how badly I might have been treated. The only thing that has any bearing over my life experience, is how I have chosen to respond. Of course, half of those choices were made without my being even vaguely aware that I was choosing, or even that I had a choice. It is no wonder then that I ended up so completely lost and in trouble. The answers are inside of us. Not in the hands of parents, teachers, doctors, healers, religious orders, cults, clubs, communities… anywhere people go to find answers, or to simply huddle together in the safety of likeness. Go inside and work out for yourself why you are here and who you truly are.

Any of those four initial wounds can knock us off track. They distort our ability to see clearly and to find our way in life. They set us on a different path from the one we planned to walk. They leave us vulnerable, as we step away from our authenticity. We learn, or choose to believe, that it is not safe or acceptable to be ourselves and so we protect ourselves by the donning of masks. We calm ourselves and sooth our wounds in invisible ways. The masks that we have come to understand make us acceptable to those whose approval and support we crave, become in fact the prisons from which we are held apart from the world that we should be living in. Behind these masks lie our vulnerabilities. We wear them like shields to protect ourselves from further harm, all the while calming and soothing our fears the best way we can, in secrecy.

Typically, there are four shields and five calming/soothing mechanisms we can adopt. They can be utilised in any combination, separately, or in conjunction with one another: Shields include, but are not limited to: Power, Perfectionism, Attitude and Invisibility.

Calming/soothing can take the form of:

- Substances (alcohol/drugs that we use to numb our feelings or seek spiritual enlightenment in the wrong place);
- Sex (multiple partners, relationships, or friendships whereby we seek outside validation of our worth and acceptability);
- Food (I separate this from substances because it is essential to life and is therefore a somewhat different construct. We might starve to achieve a thin acceptable body or we might overeat to become invisible as I did);
- Work (see how busy and important I am, no one will pick on the loyal hard working servant, the Service to the School girl);
- Social media (we can voice our opinions in virtual anonymity. Texting allows us to be involved without commitment or exposure. Games and gaming allow us to choose our reactions without having to expose ourselves. Don't like the outcome – we reset the game).

It can all become as convoluted and as complex as we choose to make it. It does however become a bit of a self-fulfilling prophesy. We feel unworthy and so we hide out pretending to be something else, thereby confirming our unworthiness. All the while we calm and sooth ourselves and say "there, there, it's all ok." So it is, until it no longer is and we hit a crisis point as our way of being becomes unsustainable; then change becomes inevitable.

Let's look at these shields we hide behind.

Power – those who are in positions of power and great authority are rarely challenged. They garner acceptance and are often actually revered by the masses. There is massive protection in hiding behind a mask of power. How many people will march into the CEO's office and call him out on his bullshit, or question his authority? Not many, because he has the power to make your life miserable, he can even threaten your livelihood. So, his wounds remain safely hidden behind his mask/shield and no one can get close enough to hurt him.

Think back to the CEO I worked with at the rehab centre. He hid his vulnerability, the fact that he wanted to be an artist and not a corporate mogul. He felt he was thus unacceptable to his family, plus he felt responsible for taking all the joy out of living (because his big sister told him it was so). He hid behind his powerful position, did what was expected of him and donned the appropriate mask.

It wasn't a problem, until it became a problem for him. Remember that everything craves resonance and he was living out of balance with his life's purpose. The resulting disharmony was causing a state of great distress. His printing plates were slightly out of register and his views on life were blurry at best. His authentic self was crying out to be heard, but he was wracked with irrational guilt and so he started dulling his pain. Calming and soothing himself with alcohol. It wasn't long before his drinking got the better of him and it became a real problem. In rehab, I was able to reconnect him with his authentic self and show him a snippet of his life plan. The rest was up to him, but at the very least his mask had slipped and he had glimpsed what was behind it.

Perfectionism – anyone have someone in their lives who has, if not the biggest home, then almost certainly the most perfectly maintained one? Every blade of grass stands to attention, every flower in the garden is picture perfect. The windows are always bright and shiny clean, letting in healthy, wholesome sunshine and providing just the right amount of warmth.

The furniture is always immaculately polished and neatly arranged for maximum comfort. The kitchen is a show piece and all meals are perfectly balanced and healthy. The children are always well dressed and tidy, never too noisy, and they achieve fantastic results at school. The parents wear the latest designer gear and the mother's makeup is always perfectly applied. There's not a hair out of place on any head in that house. Even the well-mannered dog is perfectly groomed, nails trimmed and has a shiny, wet nose.

Who among the ladies that lunch will tackle this woman, will scratch beneath the surface of her perfect exterior? She purports herself as the example for all others to strive toward, knowing that they will inevitably fall short of her unrealistic standards. She sits safely behind her mask of perfectionism, untouchable in any way. She is the chairwoman of the PTA, the go-to person for a charitable foundation. There are just no limits to her altruism. But on the inside, she is frightened silly that someone might discover how wholly unworthy she really feels; might even uncover the fact that her uncle did bad things to her when she was a child. Possibly she doesn't even remember what made her this way, but she has a driving need to not show any cracks. Her mask and her calming/soothing mechanisms might be the same, and the need to maintain a perfect life is just exhausting. Chasing perfectionism is an impossible task, since there is no such thing in the first place. I mean what is perfect, and according to whom?

Attitude – We've all come across someone who has attitude with a capital A. Perhaps they are the gregarious over-jolly, life and soul of the party people, who lead the social circle and bring the thunder to every gathering. Perhaps they are the overtly angry people who wear a threatening force field around themselves that literally repels people away from them.

They may be the bloody-minded argumentative types who are just so exhausting to be around. They will beat you to death with their opinions, refusing to stop until you are either bleeding from your ears, or you acknowledge their innate rightness and flee. People with such massive attitudes are so completely safe behind their shields, because others are either intimidated by them or, they are untouchable by virtue of their enormous energy.

How many of these jolly people need a shot of something soothing, a tranquiliser, a drink perhaps, maybe a joint in order to quell their crippling anxiety, just to get themselves to the party in the first place? How many of those angry women are starving themselves or are overeating in secret to fill the void in their lives where love and acceptance should be? How many of those argumentative folks would really love nothing more than to be held and rocked and comforted, and have someone else make all the decisions for a while? Some of them hide out in social media or gaming where the game designers have already preselected everything for them; or they cut themselves to cope with their pain.

Invisibility – Lastly, we have the shield of invisibility. We starve ourselves gorgeous, we eat ourselves out of sight, we drink ourselves bold, we live to serve, and your wish is our command. If we blindly give you what you want without question, then you won't look too closely at us and won't see how badly damaged and broken we really are.

We hide in plain sight pretending to be someone other than who we truly are, internally responding to every trigger from every situation. We take our cues from everyone we meet, who let us know in no uncertain terms how they expect us to be. We become people pleasing doormats and it is exhausting beyond belief. If you want to be my friend, I need you to always take second spot – okay I can do that. If you want to be in this club you have to follow my rules no matter how you feel – okay I can do that. If you want to work here you have to do exactly as you are told without question or pause – okay I can do that. If you want to be in this relationship, I don't want to know that you are even here, so make my life comfortable and don't ask for anything other than what you are given, and be grateful you even get that – okay I can do that too. It isn't a problem, until the day you think to yourself, but I don't really want to do that anymore.

Chapter 41

The final straw

The final straw came from one of my closest friends, my confidante, my person. The one I would have called to help me bury the body if I had ever acted out on my seething inner rage. I can only conclude after almost two years of intense grieving and soul searching, that our souls must be indelibly connected, for only a true soul connection would have the temerity to treat me as she did. I wish her nothing but joy and happiness in her life, although our friendship has been destroyed. I don't know if we will ever reconnect, or if I will even want to, but for now, I have finally learned to say No!

I was working with a coach to try and resolve some difficulties I was having adjusting to living with someone I had previously chosen to leave. All the reasons I had left Husband in the first place were still at play. Even with a different relationship dynamic, I was really struggling not to feel claustrophobic and invisible in this new set up.

My coach was able to help me see that there were two types of people: A-frame people and H-frame people. When an A-frame person is feeling vulnerable their instinct is to lean in. Hopefully they are dealing with another A-frame person who will lean in too and they can be mutually supportive. H-frame people are more inclined to be self-sufficient and don't need others to support them. They work it out for themselves, or preferably they don't take things on in the first place.

If an A-frame leans in towards an H-frame, the H-frame, who is all about self-preservation and self-interest, will simply lean away. This takes care of their own needs very successfully, but it leaves the A-frame hanging out on a limb, unfulfilled and insecure. There is nothing wrong with being either type, but you can see quite clearly how this might give rise to conflict, hurt and misunderstanding. A disconnect between two such different people is not a personal slight or affront, it is a straightforward personality clash, a challenge to be dealt with, or not.

I do believe that two such differing personality styles can live in harmony, but it requires a concerted effort and a willingness to communicate by both parties. Communication was never a strong feature in our relationship and I guess that is why we continue to struggle in close proximity. It isn't easy for either of us. Some days with ex-Husband I am reminded of my two grumpy old dogs who squabbled every day of their lives but were as close as two souls could be.

As part of our coaching conversation, we spoke about the necessity for self-care and the responsibility we all have for making ourselves feel good, for our own well-being and sense of self-worth. This led quite naturally, as it so often does in our superficial world, to the question of my weight. Anyone who is overweight is automatically seen to be uncaring of their body and self, somehow diminished in value by their supposed inability to do the right thing. Because I still spend most of my waking hours in agony, struggling to breathe and exercise is something I only dream about longingly, we decided to focus on the eating aspect.

Having tried every eating plan known to mankind, I had little hope. Also, I was disinclined to allow food to be a key player in my life, but I thought I would hear her out as she had been quite successful in helping me resolve other issues. She put forward the suggestion that I might be suffering from a food addiction. The suggestion didn't resonate with me at all. I am not unfamiliar with the addiction struggle having worked with so many addicted people in the past. I am also very aware of my own addictive tendencies.

This is why I am loath to take any medication unless absolutely necessary, and I have a strict two drinks policy. Plus, I never have even one drink on more than three consecutive days. My sister and her partner had once come to stay with me and every day after work I would be greeted with an ice-cold gin and tonic. By the third day I was shocked to find that I was ready to go home for my drink at lunchtime! I put an immediate stop to that. Could it be possible that someone so self-aware might be sitting on a hidden addiction problem? I doubted it, but I always did my due diligence with anything I was diagnosed with, so I decided to go on a journey of exploration with her, even if only to discount it once and for all.

I wasn't comfortable with the label and I decided to run it past my good friend. She had studied psychology and I trusted her opinion. I decided to share with her some of what I had been working on with the coach, and threw in a light hearted reference to the subject of food addiction, fully expecting her to say something along the lines of, "Don't be ridiculous, anyone who knows you knows that can't possibly be true."

She said nothing at the time, and we moved on with our conversation. Then she inexplicably stopped speaking to me. Her silence went on for months and I really wanted to tackle her, but I had been schooled by another friend about respecting boundaries. She was learning to put boundaries in place with some inappropriate work colleagues and she had discoursed quite passionately about it being disrespectful to overstep another person's boundaries. I elected to let it lie. In the interim I had worked with the coach and we ended up totally dismissing the idea of a food addiction. Much relieved, I decided to once again stop looking for answers and to just try and be happy instead.

I really missed my friend, but I felt like a child who had been sent to Coventry. I was bound until she decided I was done being punished. Our families spent some time together during this silent hiatus and the tension and stress of being largely ignored whilst in her company was unbearable. Then one day out of the blue, she made contact to repair the breach between us. I really wanted to know what had caused this hiatus and so I invited her right over.

It transpired that she had decided I had been lying to her about being ill for the whole thirty odd years of our friendship to hide the shameful fact of my addiction. She had given the matter much consideration and had concluded that the evidence of my addiction had been there all along. She was angry at being taken for a fool and felt I owed her an apology. I was stunned! If I live to be a hundred years old, I doubt I will ever know how she came to that conclusion. Things got pretty heated and we shouted at one another for a while and ended up hugging. She said she had made a mistake and she would never judge me again. I was so happy to have my friend back in my life. I was elated.

However, when I went to bed that night, I replayed the exact words of our conversation over and over and over again in my mind. I examined the energy of the transaction and I heard it not through the relief of someone desperate to be loved and accepted, or through the filter of a second-rate, people pleasing doormat, who, as I had been taught my entire life, should be grateful for anyone who wanted to be with me, but through my own true soul.

I had been judged harshly, incorrectly and unfairly and I had been punished for almost six months. Now that she was ready to move on, I was expected to carry on like it had never happened. I could not do that. When trust is shattered, it takes tremendous effort to rebuild it and I didn't have it in me. It takes all of my energy just to get through the day. I had so much to deal with and there was nothing left over.

Anyone or anything that took away from me or added to my burden had to be let go. I felt as though I was fighting for my life, locked in a battle for self-preservation. Saying no became a moral imperative.

I went into a cycle of grieving so deep and so profound I sometimes wondered whether I would ever recover. I cried every day and every night for almost two years. I mourned the loss of the friendship harder than I had mourned anything else in my life. I consulted my coach and a therapist to try and make sense of it all, and to find any way to be at peace with what I felt to be a huge betrayal. I wanted to know if I could ever find my way back to this friendship.

Both professionals recommended that for my own well-being and peace of mind, I step away. Looking back, I still marvel at how long it took me to find my own worth in this situation. I regret putting someone else's well-being above my own. I regret my passive behaviour in the name of consideration. I regret not standing up for myself against her unkindness and not prioritising me. I understand that an error in judgement is just that, an error, a lapse, a misunderstanding, a mistake, we all make them.

I also understand that by electing not to seek to clarify, correct and resolve a situation, that error becomes a choice. We had both made poor choices. She chose to stay in her judgement and condemnation of me, and by deciding to let an untenable situation stand for so long, I unwittingly chose to accept it. I have to own my part in the dissolution of our friendship. I regret not fighting harder for us before it was too late.

My worth is no longer subject to interpretation by anyone else, or dependant on anyone else's opinion of me. How others see me or think about me is truly of no concern to me. Their opinions have no bearing on my life. If I have to stand alone for the rest of my life, I would choose that rather than subject myself to the harsh scrutiny and judgement of others. Certain relationships have, of necessity, been let go and others have been moderated. I have become adept at stepping back from people and situations that seek to minimise me.

I am no longer available for the roles of doormat and punching bag. I am not available to be the butt of snide comments and judgements. The wonderful thing about this is that I have begun to attract new people into my life. People who see all of me, including my warts, my weight, my quirks, my strengths, my weaknesses, my frailties and above all, my open heart. People who see what is right with me and they celebrate that. People who, when I'm struggling, stand beside me without judgement until I'm strong again. People who do not require me to be anything other than who and what I am; and I have finally learned to say No!

Using meditation, hypnosis and Inner Tuition it is possible to explore previous incarnations. If there is something that affects you profoundly and you cannot find a way to understand it, it is possible that you are playing out some unfinished business from a prior lifetime. If you have a limiting belief that makes no sense to you, it may be from a previous lifetime too.

Kinesiologists can pick this up with muscle testing, but they cannot give you a true understanding. If you want to really know the details and unpack it properly, you need to do the journey work. There are many disciplines that use hallucinogenic substances to achieve these journeys. That is not necessary at all. In the hands of a skilled facilitator you can do this journey work without aids; and with self-discipline and practice, you can do the work by yourself using only your breath as the tool to get you there.

It is a fascinating process and I have managed to reach a profound understanding of many situations and relationships using these techniques. As always though, understanding on its own is insufficient to affect a change in your life. You need to take some action utilising the new knowledge and insight you have gained if you wish to achieve lasting change.

Grief is one of the most powerful emotions a human can experience. Grief is not only related to death. One can grieve loss of circumstances, skills, opportunities, faculties… indeed anything that once was and is no more; or anything that should have been and wasn't. My life was consumed by grief. A lot of what I thought was repressed anger, was in reality grief.

The depression the medical world kept alluding to, that I had refuted at every turn, knowing instinctively I was not depressed, was in fact a deep, soul level sadness. I grieved for the childhood I wished I'd had, for my loss of innocence, for my ability to earn a living, for friendships I had lost, for opportunities to learn that I was denied, for my parents, my soul animals, my fully functional brain, my able body, my home, my independence; it was a very long list.

Grief will always find a way. It has to, simply because it is so powerful. The only way to grieve properly is to allow yourself to acknowledge your feelings and to give yourself permission to feel them, no matter how painful, or how afraid you are that they will consume you. By allowing them airspace, you validate those feelings and that affords them the opportunity to transmute to a deeper understanding, or an acceptance and hopefully you will finally come to a place of being at peace with them. Grief can act as a catalyst for great change. Similarly, repressed grief can and will close your life down until you are unrecognisable even to yourself. The longer you resist grieving, the harder it will be to express it. Seek help if you must, call a friend, join a grief group, find a therapist, but allow your grief expression so that you can learn to live again, fully, authentically and unfettered.

People talk about getting over grief. I don't believe one can ever get over something so profound, but you can find a way to move forward in your life again in spite of the grief and the loss. If you do not allow yourself to grieve however, it will consume you. Far better to do the hard work so that the circumstances that caused you such grief, can be transmuted to yet another inert cave painting on the wall of your life's story, rather than a three headed monster that consumes you and threatens your well-being and peace of mind.

I worked with a wonderfully courageous lady in rehab. Her young teenage son had died tragically in a freak accident that should never have happened. The intensity of her feelings threatened to stop her breath and she simply could not allow herself to grieve. She plastered over her feelings and continued with her life, throwing herself into work with great gusto.

Her colleagues and friends praised her stoicism and her courage. After work however, she went home and sat still in her chair, staring at the walls until she went to bed. She could not allow herself to enjoy anything because her beautiful son could not enjoy it with her. She decided that feeling joy or happiness was to deny the horror of his loss and would be disrespectful to his memory. She punished herself by denying what she felt and she literally froze in her grief, willing herself to die too. Eventually she began to comfort and sooth herself with alcohol. It wasn't long before her world imploded and she was without a job. She then had nothing but her grief to fill her days. The image I was given for her when I scanned her body was the song, "Take me out to the ball game, take me out to the park…"

After much hard work in rehab, she allowed her feelings free rein and came to accept that her dynamic young son would not have wanted her to live frozen because of him, he would want her to live as fully as she could for both of them. I suggested she build a little alter in one corner of her home where she might place candles and pictures of her son, perhaps something personal of his that he had loved, whatever felt right to her. That would give her a focal point for her grief and she could stop at the end of every day and chat to him, filling him in on all the wonderful things she had done that day. She could take his energy, his memory, out to the ball game and come home and share the experience with him. This would allow her to be free for the rest of the day to live fully whilst still honouring his memory. Slowly she could come back to life. I really hope she made the decision to do so.

Chapter 42

The body speaks

There are many books available that discuss how dis-ease and imbalance in one's life might show up as physical symptoms. They don't always say exactly the same thing, but as always, I believe we need to work out for ourselves the language of our own Inner Tuition. With permission, I have included this extract from the Inner Tuition manual. If this differs from your understanding, that is absolutely fine. I have found this very useful in my work with myself and with clients. This doesn't mean that every time you have a twinge or a pain it is indicative of a major blockage or imbalance in your life. Sometimes you do just catch a cold, bump your head or slam your fingers in the car door. Recurrence or patterns of problems however, are an indication that closer scrutiny is indicated.

Please note that any references to masculine and feminine energy do not pertain to males and females or any iteration of those gender stereotypes. Masculine energy embodies the qualities of control, direction, logic, linear thinking, assertiveness, assessing, indoctrination. Think military, banking, governing bodies, science, medicine and I'm sure you can see the patterns inherent in masculine energy. Our entire societal structure is based on masculine principles.

Feminine energy on the other hand is inclined towards, nurturing, allowing, supporting, encouraging and caring. Our planet is in the midst of a shift towards the feminine energy. As the balance of power is shifting, more than ever, we need to find new ways of managing our resources, of relating to one another, of redressing the utter imbalance in people's living conditions and opportunities, and of nurturing our planet.

Change is always challenging and on such a grand scale it is bound to create ripples and in some cases tsunamis, as those not quite ready to embrace the change feel ever threatened and push back with a desperation born of fear. The early adopters will be out there finding creative solutions to problems created by a linear thinking society. More and more people are becoming conscious of their heart connections and the huge influx of differently abled children and souls is creating a moral imperative to move towards kindness, acceptance and love as a way of life. Once again, I digress, my apologies. Back to the language of the body.

The left side of the body represents Yin energy. Dis-ease or discomfort on the left side of the body may well relate to issues with the female or feminine influences in our lives, being mother, sister, wife, aunt, daughter, female friends or colleagues, and so on. Or we may be holding back our intuition, or possibly we are not allowing ourselves to express our caring, nurturing energy. In women, they may have conflicting feelings regarding their own femininity. In a man, it could be to do with his beliefs about women in general, or his own feminine energy. For either sex, the left side is also representative of the spiritual side of our nature.

The right side of the body represents Yang energy. Dis-ease or discomfort on this side of the body may relate to the male or masculine influences in our lives, such as father, brother, son, husband, male friends or colleagues. The Yang energy relates to issues of career, how we move forward in life, and what we do in the world. In a man it could relate to his beliefs about himself as a man, or his masculinity. In women, it could be to do with negative beliefs held about men in general, or about her own masculine energy. It is our logical, linear thinking, assertive nature that deals with money, success, prosperity, and how we relate to the outside world.

Every part of the body can be used to indicate something specific and it is helpful to have more understanding of this in our quest to transform our consciousness and heal our lives.

Head

The head is the control centre for the whole body and issues the commands which run the body. Problems with the head all relate to issues of self. Repeated head injuries could indicate a frustration with our self and with our situation in life. If we feel inadequate, we can try too hard in life and this can lead to us experiencing headaches. Low self-esteem might cause us to criticize ourselves and drive ourselves too hard until we experience migraines. If we are too much in our head, worrying, thinking, cogitating all the time, we might give ourselves overload headaches.

I have suffered my entire adult life with debilitating migraine headaches. I had viral encephalitis when I was pregnant with my first child. I have bounced on my head more times than is healthy, either courtesy of mother, or falling off my horse, or swan diving down an embankment Humpty Dumpty style. To say I felt frustration with myself and my situation would be a gross understatement and clearly, I have suffered with low self-esteem – it is my primary karma.

Nerves

The nervous system is our alarm system. The nerves are constantly communicating messages to every part of the body. If we have a problem with a damaged nerve, it would seem that our communications have broken down. Who aren't we communicating with? What aren't we communicating? Is there something within ourselves we are not in touch with? Is our alarm system in overdrive?

Living in a constant state of nervous anticipation, waiting for the other shoe to drop, the next criticism to be levied, the next threat to my well-being literally from day one, set my nervous system into a state of disarray. Living in a state of fight or flight and seldom relaxing into rest and response, led to adrenal fatigue and exhaustion. My body forgot how to regulate its own nervous responses.

Hair

Our hair could be indicative of our thoughts and strengths. Is our hair wild, frizzy and undisciplined, lank and weak, shining and healthy, or neat and controlled? When our hair falls out it could indicate a fear that we can't cope with some aspect of our life. Constant worrying thoughts might cause our scalps to tense so much that nourishment is cut off from the roots and they die. Baldness may indicate that worry is undermining our strength or it could simply be hereditary.

Eyes

Our eyes are the windows of our soul. If someone doesn't meet our eyes we know, albeit unconsciously, that they are lying or do not believe what they are saying. When we have eye contact with someone, we are meeting them soul to soul. Not making eye contact with someone might simply be because of a cultural taboo.

- If we are near-sighted, we may fear the future.
- If we are far-sighted, we may be an outgoing personality who doesn't like looking at intimate relationships and things close to us.
- Cataracts would indicate that our future appears uncertain to us, our vision is clouded over.
- With glaucoma there is a build-up of pressure. Emotions may have been building up resulting in our only seeing a very narrow pathway ahead.

- Astigmatism suggests that our reality is, or was, quite uncomfortable so we try to distort our picture of reality.

I always had an astigmatism until my cataracts completely clouded my vision at a time in life when my future was entirely uncertain. I have come to realise that when I am being inauthentic as I still am from time to time (donning a protective mask if I am feeling overwhelmed or insecure), I struggle to make eye contact.

Ears

Our ears represent how we hear things around us. If we don't like what we hear, and we can't get away from it, we may withdraw into deafness, temporary or permanent. If we are angry or irritated by what we hear, we may develop an ear infection.

- Children who are unable to escape conflict at home or at school may develop inflammation in their ears.
- Tinnitus, which is ringing in the ears, is the mind's way of drowning out things we don't want to hear. It may also be that we are not listening to our inner voice, the voice of our Higher Self.

The tinnitus in my ears is deafening which is no wonder since I have spent my entire life avoiding my Higher Self. The ear infection I developed after my daughter was car jacked was a clear expression of something I did not want to hear and being on the left side also pointed to an issue with a female or feminine aspect in my life, as well as my feelings of inadequacy in that I, as a mother, could not protect or help my child when she was in danger.

Nose

Our nose represents our intuition and therefore our sense of who we are.

- When it gets blocked, we may not be listening to our intuition or we may feel we are not being recognized.
- A runny nose is an acceptable way to cry, if we can't express our feelings openly.
- Sneezing or blocked sinuses suggest that we are irritated by someone. Who is it? And of course, nose problems could indicate we are being nosey.

I suffered recurring sinus infections since returning to live with my ex-Husband where I found myself in a state of perpetual irritation. I really needed to work on that. I also felt perennially unrecognised.

Mouth

Our mouth is where we take nourishment in the form of food. We also express ourselves through our mouth. Mouth problems could result from speaking ill of others, bad mouthing them. Perhaps what is going on in our life is leaving a bad taste in our mouth. Our mouth is a very sensitive, intimate area and mouth ulcers could indicate that we are being eaten away by a lack of love, with lack of self-love being a major factor here.

I have always suffered from ulcers in my mouth, abscesses in my gums and a painful burning sensation in my tongue.

Teeth

We bite and chew with our teeth. They symbolize how we speak, or how we chew over a problem. Rotting or infected teeth could indicate a need to purify what we say or think. Do we gossip unkindly? Teeth are symbolic of decisions; if we have loose teeth, or aching teeth possibly we are unable to make decisions or perhaps we agonize over them. Problems with the gums indicate indecisiveness.

Having to have fourteen teeth worked on in one go could be due to all the cortisone I took throughout my misdiagnosed life, or it could very well be indicative of my being unable to make decisions about my own worthiness.

Lips

Kissing is a very intimate form of closeness and lip sores prevent this closeness. What are we sore about? Is closeness difficult for us? Do we feel guilty about enjoying so much closeness? Lips express emotions and we may have learned to hold back or keep a stiff upper lip. What are we holding back now?

Jaw

We clench our teeth in anger, clamping down on our jaw. This could indicate that we are holding on tight and controlling our feelings. We may be afraid to speak in case we change things for the worse, or maybe we are too afraid of what we might say if we let go. To release this tension, we need to be able to express our feelings honestly. If words are difficult, perhaps we could release some tension by writing our feelings down or speaking them to a pet or an inanimate object.

I have held so much tension in my jaw that I caused trigeminal neuralgia. A neurologist I consulted about the searing pain I was experiencing in my forehead and face suggested I might have a conversion disorder. That is a neurological problem with the brain's wiring that essentially leads the patient to experience symptoms that are not real. This condition used to reside in the field of psychiatry, but recent thinking has moved it to the field or neurology and it is neither testable, provable, nor treatable. My trusty physiotherapist was able to release the tension in my jaw and ease my extreme symptoms. The pain as it turned out was a recurrence of shingles – another incorrect life-limiting diagnosis dodged.

Neck

This connects our head (our thinking), with our heart (our feelings).

- A long neck might indicate a split between the body and the mind, or perhaps a desire to separate from our feelings.
- A short neck may indicate a difficulty integrating our thoughts and feelings.
- Stiff necks may indicate that we are being stubborn, inflexible or proud about something.

There is always another point of view, what might it be? When we have a pain in the neck, we should ask who or what is a pain in our neck? The answer usually is glaringly obvious.

Having twisted my neck around like an owl during the Humpty Dumpty episode I could conclude that I was trying to find another point of view.

Throat

The throat is a very sensitive area and this is where we connect with our inner guidance. Our throat blocks when we don't speak our truth, so if we frequently get a frog in the throat, or constantly need to clear it, it may be that we are not speaking our truth or are overly concerned that what we are saying will not be accepted by others.

If we swallow anger, hurt or disappointment, we may develop sore throats. What do we really want to say? Who do we need to speak to? What are we choking back, or who are we being choked by? If we are very angry and are afraid that we may say something which will lose us our job, or relationship, we may lose our voice. This is our unconscious mind trying to protect us from danger. If we could have spoken, what would we have said and to whom?

My whole life has been one large sore throat. I have choked back so much for so long. It is amazing though that since I have accepted myself and I am expressing myself more fully, my throat no longer aches or burns.

Back

Our back is our support system. It is also where we put things behind us so that we can't see them or deal with them. Who or what do we want to turn our back on? Who is on our back, and who do we want off our back?

- **Spine:** This is our backbone and can indicate how we are living with regards to our courage, stamina and assertiveness. Our Kundalini energy, which is our life force, flows through it, so if we have no backbone, we may come across as very wishy-washy. If our spine is curved or out of alignment, our life force cannot be clearly and strongly expressed.
- **Upper back:** This part of our back lies behind the heart centre and problems here indicate anger or fear that we are not being loved or emotionally supported as we would like to be. It can also indicate that we are wanting to let go of people or situations that we have been carrying. I lived for three decades with a spasm in my upper back between my shoulder blades.
- **Middle back:** This is the part behind the solar plexus, where we hold our self-esteem and self-worth. Problems here indicate that old guilts, anger and power struggles are holding us back. It is time to raise our consciousness and lift our thought patterns so that the energy can move up to the spiritual. I actually broke my back in this area. I was living under so much pressure from being inauthentic in my own life, that when I fell, my backbone literally snapped under the pressure.
- **Lower back:** This relates to how we feel supported, emotionally and financially by the universe. This is our survival area. If we feel threatened, for example we've lost our job; can't pay the mortgage; a relationship has broken down; someone we relied on is ill – our lower back will show strain. We can be outwardly secure, but still fear something will be taken away. Lower back problems indicate a need for inner security.
- **Slipped disc:** Here there is an inner conflict about a core issue. Are we pressurizing ourselves, or is someone or something outside us the problem?
- **Osteoporosis:** This is where we feel that our emotional support system is crumbling. I've had a slipped disc, been diagnosed with osteopenia (the forerunner of osteoporosis), I broke my

back, dislocated my coccyx... looking at these explanations I can't say I'm surprised that the disharmony in my life showed up in my back.

Shoulders

We carry our burdens and responsibilities on our shoulders. This is where we carry the decisions we have made for this life.

- Sloping shoulder could imply that we are not willing to shoulder responsibility or burdens.
- Square solid shoulders, however, are able to carry lots of responsibility.
- Sometimes we build overly large shoulders, which suggests that we feel we have weighty things to carry. It is a form of armouring, because we don't really want to bear it at all.
- Hunched shoulders say that we don't really want to have to deal with things.
- A frozen shoulder indicates that the flow from the heart has been frozen up with the hurt of rejection. We may feel we have been given the cold shoulder, maybe by someone dying or leaving us, or by losing our job. We can freeze up a shoulder if our womanhood or manhood has been insulted. Perhaps we want to give someone the cold shoulder? I carried so much tension in my shoulders during the retrenchment conundrum that I actually pinched a nerve. I wasn't prepared to shoulder that burden at all.

Arms

Our arms are a direct extension of our heart energy. When we open our arms to someone, we open our heart centre. So, the arms indicate the ability to reach out and embrace life, people, or situations, or how we attack it. Weapons are an extension of our arms. To carry arms suggests that we are ready to fight in order to defend ourselves, or conversely, to attack.

Elbows

Our elbows can give grace to the expression of our arms, or they can be bony and awkward. Problems here indicate difficulty changing our ideas about life. Who do we want to elbow out? Who's elbowing us out? Do we resent having to put in too much elbow grease? Tennis elbow is an inflammation of the tendon, which indicates difficulty in making moves, mental, emotional or physical. It is very painful, so perhaps we are feeling guilty about wanting to make moves?

Hands

Hands express how we handle life. With hands we give and receive, so if we have problems with our hands we can ask: are we being tight-fisted or open-handed? Are we clutching and holding on? Who is cramping our style?

- Do we have cold hands so that our heart energy doesn't reach what we are doing?
- Are our hands hot and sweaty, indicating that we're pouring too much emotion into what we are doing? Our hands touch, stroke and applaud. How do we feel about doing these things?
- Skin rashes indicate how we feel we are handling an issue; do we feel good (attractive) about how we are dealing with it?

Fingers

Fingers express how we deal with the details of life

For years I had itchy, acidic rashes in the creases of my elbows and on my hands and fingers.

Chest

Our chest protects our heart centre which houses our feelings and emotions, our secrets, longings, hopes and desires. So how do we present ourselves to the world? We may puff out our chests to pretend we are more powerful than we feel; or put on a good front to cover our inadequacies. We may be closed-chested and afraid to open our hearts, or we may build powerful chests to armour our vulnerable hearts.

Lungs

Our lungs indicate our ability to breathe freely or to breathe for ourselves. They express our ability to be independent and self-assured. Problems indicate that we daren't breathe because we are afraid of life, or because we are controlled or dominated by someone.

- Asthma might indicate that we are dependent on someone looking after us, and that we are afraid to breathe for ourselves. Are we emotionally smothered by someone? We may have unexpressed grief which may be many lives deep.
- A cough suggests irritation. What do we want to get off our chest? What do we want to express?

During each of the last three years before the retrenchment conundrum, I spent a period in hospital with protracted asthma attacks. I had an unrelenting cough for years and years; and one of my earliest symptoms was bronchitis and pleurisy that both affect the lungs.

Breasts

Women nurture with their breasts. Problems here might indicate a tendency to over-nurture, perhaps wanting to prove our womanhood or femininity, or that we are a good mother. Or we may want to keep people dependent on us so that they won't leave us. We are compensating for the part of us that feels unnurtured. We may also have problems in this area because we feel we ought to nurture others and we don't want to. Either way, cancer of the breast indicates that our needs are not being met, as we feel our role is to meet the needs of others. Breasts are also the sexual symbol of our womanhood, and conflicts about how we feel as a sexual woman can be expressed in this area of the body.

- The left breast expresses our feelings about being a woman, wife or mother, and our distress that our needs in this area are not being met.
- The right breast expresses our conflicts in life as a woman.

Repeated mastitis in my right breast while breastfeeding seems reasonable reading the above; as do the recurrent abscesses in my left breast.

Heart

If our heart is open, we forgive hurts and slights easily and we are open to the joy of life. However, if we hold on to old hurts and harden or clamp down on our heart, we create the conditions for heart attacks.

- Angina indicates that we are squeezing our heart with hurt, or perhaps we feel it is too dangerous to be loved.
- High blood pressure shows that we are feeling under emotional pressure from past hurts, or that we feel unloved and want more love.

I suffer with high blood pressure, and my Dad had angina.

Solar plexus

This is where we hold our gut feeling. Our gut relates to personal courage and our ability to connect interpersonally. This is the area where we hold our feelings of self-worth, confidence and self-esteem. It is our power centre.

Stomach

This is where we digest ideas. How do we stomach the things in our life?

- When we get an upset stomach, is there someone or something we can't stomach? Perhaps we can't stomach the idea of something happening?
- When we feel empty of love, we may try to stuff ourselves with a love substitute being food, especially sugar. This is the basis of obesity.
- The opposite is anorexia, where we try to control our feelings of not being loved, by not letting food (love) in.
- With bulimia there is a feeling of desperation. Our confidence and self-esteem are so low that it becomes self-loathing. We stuff ourselves with food (love), and then reject it by being sick. Underneath we are crying out to be loved, nourished and accepted.
- If we have an ulcer, we can ask what's eating away at us. Is it resentment, hurt, bitter thoughts?

My diagnosis with SIBO Small Intestinal Bacterial Overgrowth seems pertinent in this area. The confluence of negative feelings I have harboured for almost my entire existence could most likely have given rise to rampant growth of dangerous bacteria.

Gall bladder

If we have a problem here, we have usually felt unloved or unvalued in life. When we feel resentful and bitter this may eventually crystallize into a stone.

Liver

The liver is the seat of deep emotions and this is where we hold primitive anger. Problems here indicate that our liver can't cope with all our negative emotions, and we need to relax and harmonize our life, especially our relationships.

Kidneys

Our kidneys filter and cleanse emotions and ideas. That which we no longer need is released. Kidney problems indicate that we are holding on to old emotional patterns. Old griefs and angers we have never been able to express, crystallize here and form stones. When they pass, we have been able, at one level, to let the pain go.

Makes sense of the kidney stone problem doesn't it? I was lying on the gurney outside the radiology department waiting for my CT scan when the doctor who first mis-diagnosed me with lupus walked by. Do you think Upstairs was trying to show me what anger I needed to let go of? This guy also showed up at two restaurants I was at in the following month or two. I got it, I processed it, I let it go. I no longer hate him, or most unreasonably hold him accountable for derailing my life. I made all the choices that got me to that junction and I am so much better off for releasing that anger.

Bladder

The purpose of the bladder is to release old emotions. Problems here suggest we are holding onto old feelings. Cystitis often occurs when we are feeling negative towards our partner or are holding onto deep fears which we can't express.

Bowels

The purpose of the bowels is to eliminate old ideas, concepts, thinking patterns and beliefs.

- When we have a feeling of insecurity, we try to control life, so we hang on to the old worries and problems and become constipated. We cannot forgive and forget because we are frightened to change.
- Diarrhoea indicates that we want to get rid of things quickly, without looking at, and learning from what is presented to us. Alternatively, we may be afraid and wanting to run away.

Fear of change literally twisted my gut.

Hips

Hips express our mobility, adaptability, and freedom in life. Old people who see nowhere to move forward to often fall and break a hip.

Throughout the period of reclaiming my wounded inner child my hips have been frozen, necessitating weekly physiotherapy.

Womb

This is the inner core of our being where we bring forth new life; so, problems here might indicate problems with new concepts. New ideas from the creative mind take root and develop here. Problems here come from the fears we hold about the new. Are we afraid of pregnancy or birth? Will we be a good mother? Do we really want to be tied down with children or with a new business or a new idea? When our children grow up, do we feel useless, redundant? What does life hold for us now?

When my daughters left together for the UK, I went through a complete and sudden menopause. My menstrual cycle stopped without drama or symptom. I had identified my worth as a woman by my ability to be a good mother and without my children, I simply ceased to feel relevant in my own life.

Vagina

This is our channel of creativity, through which the new seed is planted. Problems might occur here when our creativity is frustrated or we have an emotional block about sex, anger with our partner, guilt about our sexuality, or fear of invasion or deep intimacy.

Prostate

This is closely linked to sexual power which in turn may relateto a sense of confidence and personal power in men. Men enter a retirement period and they may feel confused about their role in life. Who are they and what is their function without their job? At the same time, they may be afraid that they will become sexually impotent since they have been rendered impotent / powerless in business and they fear this as a possibly in their family life.

Testicles

A man's hidden sexual fears are held here. Men may be afraid of losing their sexuality, their potency, their masculinity, their very manhood. They may be feeling emasculated.

Legs & feet

When they are strong, we can stand up for our rights and we have the power to step towards our goals. If our legs are weak, we may feel we don't have a leg to stand on. If we keep injuring our legs, we are possibly feeling undermined or are not moving in the right direction. We could also ask ourselves: who do we want to kick, or perhaps what do we want to run away from?

Since living back with ex-Husband, I have had tremendous pain in my legs, inflammation in my tendons and connective tissue. I struggle to stand and walk. Although he is extremely generous, I feel unable to support myself financially, and losing my independence has left me feeling like I don't have a leg to stand on.

Thighs

Our thighs protect our sexuality, our masculine or feminine nature. We also hold here deep emotions from our past, or deep inner fears.

Knees

Knee problems often indicate a stubborn refusal to bend to authority. On the other hand, if we are too ready to kneel and humble ourselves, we could be indicating a fear of authority, or fear of facing something or someone. Our knees tremble and buckle under us when we are afraid.

Ankles

Our ankles support us and give us flexibility to move in whichever direction we choose. Bruised, sprained or twisted ankles might indicate we don't feel supported. Perhaps we need to take a step in a new direction or we feel we can't cope in a new direction without more support. A broken ankle suggests a much deeper conflict about the direction we move in, especially if our support system has been withdrawn.

Feet

These indicate our foundation. We are solid and independent when we can stand on our own two feet; then we can put our foot down. It is with our feet that we step forward in life. If we have cold feet, it literally means we are afraid of moving forward. Foot problems suggest that we feel dependent or are not sure which direction to go in.

Having damaged tendons in my right foot, and sprained and broken toes on both feet multiple times I think it's fair to say I have issues with starting out in a new direction.

Heels

What are you being a heel about? Or who is being a heel to you? Our Achilles tendon is our weak spot, so what do you feel vulnerable about?

Toes

These indicate the minor details in life. Do we understand and cope with the small things? Toes help us stay balanced. Do little things knock us off balance? We pull back or curl up our toes as a way of withdrawing from life. What is it we don't want to deal with?

Remember that just because you have a twinge in some area of your body, that doesn't necessarily mean you have a life crisis lurking. Repeated problems in a specific area can certainly indicate that there might be something that is out of balance in your life. When seeking answers however, the body holds lots of information for you to ponder and examine.

Chapter 43

Letting go

Trauma plays out in a number of different ways in our lives. In a very crude cliff notes version of so many articles I have read: the brain has a three-way response system built in, the reptilian brain; the limbic brain; and the neocortex.

The reptilian brain

The most primitive part of our brain, the reptilian brain, is part of our subconscious mind. It controls the body's vital functions such as heart rate, breathing, body temperature and balance. Our reptilian brain includes the brainstem and the cerebellum. It is reliable but tends to be somewhat rigid and compulsive. It will therefore imprint trauma with a permanence that will dominate its future. It understands images rather than language, which is why visualisation is such a useful tool for dealing with problems rooted in this area. This part of the brain dominates at birth.

The limbic brain

The limbic brain is involved in learning, memory and emotion. It records memories of behaviours that resulted in either agreeable or disagreeable experiences. This is why repetition is such a powerful tool when teaching children, or indeed any age group. A positive experience repeated often will create a positive record. The same is true of a negative or disagreeable experience. The limbic brain is responsible for us feeling emotions such as excitement, pleasure, anger, fear, sadness, joy, disgust, shame and so on. The main structures of the limbic brain are the hippocampus, the amygdala, and the hypothalamus. The limbic brain is the seat of our values and exerts a strong influence on our behaviour.

The neocortex

The neocortex with its two large cerebral hemispheres, is where we process conscious thought and self-awareness. It is also where we develop language, abstract thought, imagination, and problem solving. It has an almost infinite learning ability. Logical thinking though, is not apparent until around the age of six or seven. This is why you will never win an argument with a toddler. They simply lack the cognitive ability to reason and they will hit you with a wall of emotion (limbic response) to make their position know to you.

If we experience an occasional trauma, our brain will trigger an emotional response that in essence releases or minimises the effects of the trauma. Tears are a good way of releasing trauma. Ongoing painful experiences though, can actually engrave new circuits in the brain. When this happens, we become primed to feel trauma in response to something that another person might not even notice. This hypersensitivity can be dangerous, but it does support the theory that once a core wound is set up in childhood, it creates an overly sensitive filter, shaping subsequent events.

If we are harbouring a childhood wound and we experience something similar as an adult, both the new and the childhood responses are triggered, thus magnifying the experience. If we do not work with our original trauma, because we are either unaware it is there, or we have been taught to inhibit ourselves to be found acceptable to our caretakers or teachers, we learn to numb out or bury the response. This unresolved emotion that cannot be expressed as, for example, grief, might well lead to acting out or acting in, and the accompanying behavioural problems.

We are set up for a lifetime of over-reacting to triggers that to an emotionally healthy person may in fact be totally insignificant. Since energy cannot be destroyed, and we have not allowed this energy (these emotions) to be transmuted to understanding, they are repressed and stored safely for us by our shadow self.

It is a common misconception that our shadow side is something to be denied and is comprised of our basest nature. We have an inherent, if irrational fear that by examining it we might unleash our inner axe murderer. In reality, our shadow is our greatest ally. It holds all the pieces of ourselves that we are not willing to face. We may have decided as a toddler that we needed to be someone or something else in order to be acceptable to those whose approval we sought. This led to us quashing our natural authentic self and the subsequent donning of masks.

Either we didn't feel safe to be fully us, or the desire for approval was stronger than our sense of self, or perhaps something was simply too painful to deal with. Whatever it was that we felt we could not handle, together with all the hidden aspects of ourselves (some of which we may not even be aware we have hidden away) are kept preserved and safe. When the day comes that we finally admit we are out of balance in our lives and hopefully begin to do our inner journey work, our shadow holds some important information that we may need to access. It is quite natural to suppress parts of our self that we have been conditioned to believe are undesirable or incongruent with the family, group, community or affiliation we find ourselves part of. Looking at, and owning, those supposedly undesirable parts of ourselves can take a great deal of courage, but it is always a liberating experience.

I have dealt with so many people who had hidden away from the world certain experiences that they found so heinous, they could not even allow themselves to face them. The gentleman I worked with who watched his puppy being killed by his father was one of these. He buried that memory so deep in his shadow, that he didn't even remember it was there. Child victims of sexual molestation often develop intense feelings of shame and guilt and their very survival feels contingent upon them hiding the source of their shame from the world.

Instead of getting the support and care they actually needed to be able to make sense of the violation they experienced, they ended up supressing the memory. They don elaborate masks to protect themselves, ensuring no one can ever get close enough to see their shameful truth. They live in a state of perpetual imbalance and eventually this will show up somewhere in their adult lives. All calming and soothing mechanisms have the potential to harm us if our need for them consumes our reality.

At some point a problem we buried all those years ago, becomes a problem in our daily lives. In order to survive and thrive, we need to begin our healing journey. We can examine our shadow self in small incremental bites so as not to frighten ourselves, but the more we can release our shadow side, the more fully authentic we become. Remember we have a unique light pattern or light fingerprint that Upstairs uses to identify us… well our shadow distorts that light and the only way to attain enlightenment, is to embrace all the colours in our spectrum.

Understanding this helped to explain why my emotional and subsequent physical reaction to my daughters carjacking was so extreme. Every time I had felt threatened, unsafe, or powerless in the past and I hadn't dealt with it, those repressed feelings were called into play. The resulting huge reaction set off a cataclysmic emotional response quite out of balance with the actual event. It also explains why I struggled to turn off the response once I found out she was safe. All that unresolved emotion from my past, most of which I did not even know about or understand, was magnifying my response. The same understanding can be used to explain why, when my sister's partner passed away so unexpectedly, I did not have the same exaggerated response. I had no past experience of sudden bereavement associated with trauma stored in my shadow, and without that added distortion I was able to process a really difficult situation in a normal, healthy way.

Unpacking one's shadow becomes imperative when faced with unexplained physical symptoms that threaten your existence, or ongoing repetitive and similar challenges that continue to crop up. In order to bring about healing, it is necessary to lift up the rocks of your past and see what is hiding underneath them. Some experiences need nothing more than having a little light shone on them to transmute them safely out of shadow.

The simple act of acknowledgement is enough to affect the desired change. This is because when we look at them with a lifetime of collective wisdom, from the safety of an adult reality, we don't find them nearly as frightening or threatening as we did in childhood. Other aspects of us that have been buried for a long time, or have been actively denied, and especially those that we are unaware even exist, need more careful consideration once unearthed, and you may need help to deal with those.

Every part of yourself that you can reclaim, the good, the bad, and especially the ugly, helps you to become more fully authentic, more fully you. Your view on life becomes less distorted with each discovery and revelation and the more you can transmute your darkness into light, the happier you will feel, and the more in balance your life becomes.

It can be very challenging for other people in your life as you change and become a brighter, clearer version of yourself. If someone needs you to be, or act, a certain way in order to support their illusion, then your new brighter way of being may frustrate or even threaten them.

Change comes with consequences and those who need you to behave a certain way, may even stage an energetic attack on you to try and force you back to the way you were before. The only comfort you need be concerned with, is your own. If any relationship in your life requires you to be, or act in a certain way, then that relationship bears scrutiny. A truly loving relationship is one where we celebrate each other and want the best for the other person. This sentiment is articulated most eloquently by the great William Shakespeare's sonnet 116: *Love is not love which alters when it alteration finds.*

I went on an amazing course that helped me tremendously in a most surprising way. I had identified so much hidden grief and sorrow in my life and I was fully aware of how these emotions had ruled me and overshadowed much of my life's experience. I had made my peace with so much of my past and had reclaimed vast tracts of my shadow self. Yet I still suffered from so much physical pain.

I was racked with inflammation and I seemed to be at an impasse. The course I attended was aimed at using breath work to manage chronic pain. Delightfully, the use of therapy horses was part of the process. I learned about the sympathetic and the para-sympathetic nervous systems and how I could use breathing to switch from one to the other. I had spent over fifty years primarily in *fight or flight* mode and I had no idea how to get myself back into *rest and repose*. This would account for my adrenal fatigue and the resultant imbalance of my hormonal systems that made it impossible for me to lose weight.

One generally switches into the sympathetic nervous system in response to a threat. This gives you the added adrenalin needed to run away (think of the tiger in the jungle scenario, where a hasty retreat is your best chance of survival). Once safe, you switch back to your para-sympathetic nervous system, relax, and go about your business.

My reptilian brain had decided when I was born that I was not safe. That thinking was reinforced by the behaviour of my mentally ill Mother throughout my initial start in life. My limbic brain had successfully added multiple confusing layers of emotions and feelings to the mix, and by the time my neocortex had developed and I could think for myself with any clarity, certain responses had been reconfigured in my brain; I was no longer making rational, healthy connections. This distorted response left me feeling threatened all of the time, and so I stayed in sympathetic mode, ready to fight off the next person or situation that threatened me.

Simply speaking, we have five know brainwave states. There is much literature to be found on this subject, but again this is my cliff notes version.

Delta brainwaves

Delta brainwaves (.5 – 3 HZ) are generated only in the deepest of meditative states and during deep, dreamless sleep. Delta waves suspend body awareness and stimulate healing and regeneration which is why deep sleep is so essential to the healing process. This is also where we find our empathy.

Theta brainwaves

Theta brainwaves (3 – 8 HZ) occur most often when we sleep but, are also apparent in deep meditation. Theta is where we experience learning, memory and intuition. In theta, our focus is within and we are not aware of our surroundings. It is that twilight state we experience at the moment we wake or when we are drifting off to sleep. We dream in theta and we can experience vivid imagery, connect with our intuition, and access information beyond our normal conscious awareness. This is where we access our fears, troubles and nightmares.

Alpha brainwaves

Alpha brainwaves (8 – 12 HZ) are dominant in a light meditative or contemplative state where we experience quietly flowing thoughts. Alpha is where we experience being in the moment, fully present. Alpha is a resting state for the brain and helps with overall mental coordination, calmness, alertness, mind/body integration and learning.

Beta brainwaves

Beta brainwaves (12 – 38 HZ) dominate in our normal waking state of consciousness. Here we are focussed on cognitive tasks and the outside world. Beta is present when we are alert, attentive, engaged in problem solving, judgment, decision making, or focused mental activity from musing, through actively figuring something out, to new experiences, high anxiety, or excitement. This continual high frequency processing takes a tremendous amount of energy.

Gamma brainwaves

Gamma brainwaves (38 – 42 HZ) are the fastest of brain waves and relate to simultaneous processing of information from different brain areas. Gamma brainwaves pass information rapidly and quietly. The most subtle of the brainwave frequencies, the mind has to be quiet to access gamma. It is highly active when in states of universal love, altruism and the higher virtues, expanded consciousness and spirituality.

Humans when awake, are predominantly in a Beta brainwave state and this is where we do all of our neocortex thinking; that mulling and chewing over of life. It is that constant internal chatter that makes us crazy and keeps our stress levels way up. I learned that horses don't live in this state. They exist in an Alpha brainwave state. They are relaxed and at peace, they flow with the rhythm of life whilst calmly maintaining their focus.

They only go into a Beta brainwave state as a direct result of a threat. Historically horses are prey animals and so they rely on a very effective *get up and go* mechanism in order to survive. Conversely their ability to revert to a state of rest and repose on demand, has ensured the longevity of the species, and provides us with a perfect example of how to manage our responses.

To give your Beta brainwaves a workout, try this on for size. The human race is bombarded with stressful stimuli. Just watch the news or read a newspaper, see how aggressively people comment on innocent posts on social media. We are driven to achieve and succeed, and all the while our resources are under threat. We don't have enough money to get through the month; there is a flood, or a drought, famine, crop failure; our food sources are genetically modified making them unidentifiable to our DNA, and with our weakened immune systems, viruses and bacteria storm our bodies; our electricity supply is unstable, we are running out of coal; global warming, climate change, melting of the polar ice caps; pollution of our air, our water supply; species dying out, deforestation; we are reliant on hi tech equipment that exposes us to potentially harmful Wi-Fi or, the new kid in town – 5G; we have earthquakes, mud slides, tornados, tsunamis…

Almost every area of our lives is fraught with potential danger and the judgements, debates and arguments rage on. Our political leaders appear to have lost their minds and the established structures of our society are in danger of crumbling around us, and we get to see and hear all about it on a daily basis, because we are now a global village. The technology we have learned to become so reliant on for its efficiency and the opportunities it opens us up to, brings every single world event and piece of bad news singing straight to our smart phones, our tablets, our laptops, or our television sets.

That is a very small sample of the state of our world and it makes my stomach knot with anxiety just to write it. This is our daily reality and we wonder why there is such an increase in anxiety disorders, syndrome illnesses, and mental health issues. Humanity is in trouble and there is only one thing you can do to help, and that is to fix yourself as best you can and strive to become the enlightened soul you were always meant to be. I firmly believe that if we each took responsibility for our own impact on and in the world, we would raise the collective consciousness sufficiently to restore peace and prosperity. But I digress, back to the brainwaves and the horses.

I watched a film clip of a herd of horses, grazing peacefully in Alpha brainwave state. A child on a bicycle rode past their paddock making a loud noise. They switched straight into Beta brainwave mode and activated their sympathetic nervous systems. The lead horse ran to investigate the source of the danger, ears pricked, nostrils flaring, head and tail held high, he used fast, choppy movements making himself look as large and formidable as possible.

The horse designated as second in command, rounded up the rest of the herd and drove them to a corner as far away from the threat as possible. He then took up his position midway between the herd and the leader, ready to either support the leader or drive the herd to safety, whatever the lead horse determined was needed. The herd huddled together, safety in numbers, alert and ready to run, but awaiting instruction from their leaders.

Once the lead horse had determined there was no imminent danger, he lowered his head, relaxed his body language and snorted to release any pent-up energy. He actively drove the stress from his body and slowed his breathing. This put him straight back into Alpha brainwave state by engaging his parasympathetic nervous system. He went right back to rest and repose, and the rest of the herd followed suit. None of these horses held onto the fear, the feeling of being under threat. They were triggered to go on red alert, and immediately on sensing they were safe, they released their pent-up nervous energy and went back to a peaceful state of being. I was fascinated. I had read about it, heard about it even, but now I had seen it, and I finally understood it.

Next we were invited to go and spend time with the herd. We didn't engage with them, we toddled around the paddock and waited to see what they would do. Interestingly, a horse will not tolerate another horse who is not relaxed and whose energy is incongruent with the herd energy. Any horse exhibiting agitation is chased away from the herd. Once they have calmed themselves, they are welcomed back. The same thing happened with us.

I discovered that I had become terrified of horses which was unfathomable to me. Working through those feelings I discovered it was the fear of being hurt that was behind that. I already had so much pain in my body that I couldn't countenance taking on more and so I built a wall of fear around myself to protect me. The second in command horse came straight over and rudely shoved me out of the way.

I was in terrible pain, unable to stand for longer than three or four minutes without needing to sit down and having been rudely shoved aside by one horse and completely ignored by the rest, I decided there was nothing there for me. Once again, I was on the outside looking in, discounted and unwelcome...blah blah blah. I knew enough by now, to know this was an old pattern playing out from my days of distorted thinking. The facilitator spoke us through the breathing techniques used to engage our para-sympathetic nervous system, and as I clutched onto the fence for support, I regulated my breathing in line with the horses, pushing the out breath slightly longer than the in breath, and the noise in my mind quietened. The lead horse then came over and rested his head on my shoulder and I stood there just breathing and inhaling the scent of him. This triggered all the good memories I have associated with horses. I realised at the end of the exercise, that I had been standing with him unaided for almost thirty minutes and I had no pain in my legs at all.

We then did an exercise where we put ourselves into a dark state by focussing on our pain and all that we had lost in life. One by one the horses left the paddock and moved as far away from us as possible. We then changed the focus of our thinking to more pleasant experiences, and once we had achieved a state of happiness and calm, all the horses gravitated back to us.

We were congruent with their state of being and we were comfortable to be around again. The massive lesson for me in this exercise was how easily we had influenced our own state of mind. Truly that which you focus on grows. Thinking about loss, limitation and restriction, we had become an unstable energy to be avoided. Focussing on happiness, peace and calm, we attracted like energy to us. What you feed grows in strength; energy flows where thought goes.

This finally gave me an understanding of mindfulness. Be mindful of where you place your energy, for you certainly do create your own reality by the simple and often unconscious act of choosing your response. As with all new practices, the more time and effort you expend on them, the easier it becomes to accept them as an integral part of your normal daily existence. Once you are fully integrated with a way of being, you no longer need to mindfully focus on the practice, you naturally become this version of yourself and automatically behave in the desired manner.

Chapter 44

Checking in with yourself

So, how do you know what you need to look at, what aspects of yourself could bear some closer scrutiny? The answer to that is quite simple. What problem areas do you have in your life? Where are you out of balance? It is a good practice to check in with yourself at regular intervals to see how you are doing.

Meditation is one of the tools you can use to do this. Here's a meditation we often did whilst studying with Inner Tuition. In a meditative state, you take yourself to a place of great comfort to you, be it a memory of a place where you felt safe and loved, or under the shade of a massive tree in a meadow, or anywhere else you can imagine, as long as it feels good to you. You settle yourself down and invite your four etheric bodies to come and sit with you – physical, emotional, mental and spiritual.

It can be really interesting to see how these aspects of yourself show up in your imagination. Yes, of course you use your imagination to take these journeys, how else would you experience things never before encountered. Observe how each of your four etheric bodies represents themselves to you – physical, emotional, mental and spiritual. Mine often show up as cartoon characters. For others they experience them as colours; yet others hear music or sounds. You can connect through any of your senses.

Greet each of your etheric bodies and sit there together and see if any insights present themselves to you, engage with them and ask questions, you may be surprised at what you find out. You are getting to know a side of yourself previously unknow to you, remember the Hidden pane in the Johari Window?[1] It can be a wonderful experience.

The first time I did this exercise my physical body represented itself to me as the cartoon character Sad Sack, beaten down, slumped shoulders, defeated by life. My emotional body was Bambi, motherless,

1 See page 182

skittish and ready to flee from the fire. My mental body was Archimedes the owl, complete with spectacles, sitting atop a library rack, waiting patiently for me to engage with him. My spiritual body was a blue crane flying over a body of moonlit water, serene and unconcerned with the drama playing out in my life.

Often times the way these aspects of ourselves represent themselves to us can be indicative of something that needs attention. Having read my story, you can draw your own conclusions as to what my etheric bodies were trying to tell me. I know someone who says her subtle (etheric) bodies are often caught up in arguments with one another along the lines of, emotional body to mental body "Why should I do all the work, it's your responsibility." This indicates to her that it might be an idea to use her learning, her intellect, or her intuition to examine a situation, instead of simply reacting emotionally to it. If you allow yourself to have fun with it, this can be so revealing.

It is no coincidence that my etheric self showed up as cartoon characters, as did the messages I received when working in the rehab centre. I was completely stuck in my childhood and so my Spirit Guides spoke to me in a language that I could understand. As I have grown and released my past trauma, we are developing a more sophisticated language.

Another simpler way, for those of you who don't know how to meditate, is to do a self-examination in the bath. Showering or bathing is something we all do every day, so it is the perfect opportunity to reflect on our lives. Even if you are a shower junkie, I recommend a bath for this exercise. It creates a distinct intent to do the exercise and that is a powerful way to start.

The door is generally closed, locked even, affording you absolute privacy. You can light scented candles and throw essential oils in the bath to make you feel relaxed. You are submerged in water which is an excellent conductor of energy. Having made your preparations, first take a look at your *physical* well-being. Since you last checked in with yourself, how have you been eating, drinking, exercising, resting and so on. You might admit to yourself that nine cups of coffee a day is probably not a great way to serve the nutritional needs of your body.

Perhaps binge watching ten seasons of *How I Met Your Mother* instead of exercising hasn't added much to your physical well-being. Also smoking thirty cigarettes a day might not be the best way to optimise your health. Perhaps you might go in the other direction and acknowledge that denying yourself all carbohydrates is making you feel crabby and hard done by. Maybe three hours at the gym each day might be overdoing it a little. You might look at your physical needs and think you are doing just great. Well that's fantastic, you always have free will to choose, and this self-examination is between you and you alone.

If you are completely happy with your physical well-being then good job! Move on to your emotional examination. I must stress here that this is an observation exercise only. It is ***not*** a tool whereby you get to judge yourself and beat yourself up. You are simply observing where you are at in your life. Remember nothing is a problem, until it becomes a problem. So, if there was anything that, on observation, you felt uncomfortable about, you might want to look at making some different choices for yourself.

This is the place where you decide for yourself what you are prepared to change, in order to become more balanced and in harmony with yourself. This is about steady, incremental change that moves you comfortably toward a healthier way of being. Set small, attainable goals so that you build a culture of success and achievement for yourself. There's nothing more disheartening than aiming so high you have absolutely no chance of hitting the target. This is just self-defeating and you could end up feeling hopeless.

Perhaps decide that the nine-cup a day coffee habit is something you are prepared to tackle. My advice, unless you are in a major health crisis under doctor's orders (and that is not the ideal time for self-reflection by the way, that is the time for crisis management), is not to quit cold turkey. That is the fastest recipe for failure. The feelings of deprivation will likely plunge you into a crisis and will have an adverse effect on you.

Remember we are striving for balance in our lives. Imagine that you are on a seesaw at the park with your etheric physical self on the other end. Leaping off the see-saw at the bottom might seem like a good idea, but in effect, it will cause your physical self to come crashing down on the other side and will likely cause some harm which is counter-productive. This exercise, I say again, is not about the grand gesture, it is about making small incremental changes to achieve a state of balance and well-being.

Back to the coffee habit. What might be an acceptable change? Well your favourite cups are the ones first thing in the morning, after each meal, and maybe the last one at night before you turn in. That's five cups that give you pleasure. The other four are self-indulgent and might be considered excessive. So perhaps you might start there. Nature abhors a vacuum and it is essential for balance that if you take something away, you need to replace it with something else. That doesn't mean swop your coffee for extra cigarettes.

Exchange the extra (unnecessary) coffees for herbal tea or maybe even a glass of water or juice. That will help to counter the effects of the caffeine in your body and will aid in the quest for balance. No drama, no fuss, just a simple exchange of something harmful for something more beneficial, all the while relishing the important cups of coffee. If that is enough change for your first go on the self-examination journey, and you are fairly confident you can manage that, then stop there and be done with your physical self.

Talking about replacing harmful practices with more beneficial ones and nature abhorring a vacuum; here is a lovely little exercise you can do either as part of this self-assessment or better still as part of your daily rituals and routines. Fill a glass with water and hold it between your hands. State out loud, "I connect with the highest vibration of my soul and I fill this glass of water with unconditional love. And so it is." When you feel happy that your glass is brimming with the energy of that unconditional love, drink it all down and feel how it spreads through your body, taking with it the energy of your soul's highest vibration, filling you with unconditional love. What a simple statement of intent that requires no skill, no time and no resources. When anyone asks me how they can change, this is a great place to start.

Remember this bathtub assessment is an observation only and you need to prime yourself to succeed. If you think you can handle more then have a look at your exercise or sleeping habits and find another area to make new choices about. Continue as you have been without judgement, focussing only on the small incremental changes you decide to make. The only person you are accountable to is yourself. Everything else that you flagged as needing a change, will still be there next time you check in. Once you have created a culture of achievement for yourself, you will be able to tackle more challenging changes, incrementally.

Next you look at your emotional self. How have you expressed your emotions? Have you been repressing how you feel, or have you perhaps been over-reacting? Was it prudent and in your best interests to have shouted at your manager in frustration today? Perhaps not. A healthier option might have been to find a different way to diffuse the situation. That doesn't mean your feelings are not valid, but do remember that just because you feel something, doesn't mean you have to express it immediately.

It is perfectly acceptable, preferable even, that you take time out to reflect on why you felt so triggered by a situation. Own your feelings and try to find out how you might make a different choice if the same situation presented itself again. A manager acting like a bully is not something you should ever have to tolerate. Facing them down head-on though, will add nothing to your cause and you may be seen as a subordinate with a bad attitude. Human Resources should be staff-focussed in an office situation and can be appealed to for arbitration in such matters. Likewise, a teacher being inappropriate with a student can be sidestepped and a student council member might be approached instead. Reacting to a triggered emotion is seldom, if ever, beneficial in the long run. It is better to try and understand why you were triggered in the first place.

If you have no specific emotional problem, but you are maybe feeling a little blue, then what better place than in the privacy of your bath to allow your feelings expression, perhaps allow some tears to flow. Remember tears transmute energy from one state to another. Another example of emotional health is that you might be feeling on top of the world, but you have been taught to repress your emotions. Well singing in the bath is a well-recognised way of expressing joy too. Either way, find one small thing that you can make a different choice about and commit to that. You will feel better for having done so.

I had a wonderful client who came to me complaining that she felt emotionally dead. She had lost the ability to feel anything. She was as jumpy as a snake and was very uncomfortable. There were clearly some deep-seated issues, but she was absolutely not open to working with them, or to seeing a therapist, or getting medical treatment. She was at the very beginning stage of her journey, testing the waters to see what might happen if she dared to admit there might be a problem. This is a delicate stage indeed and is often underpinned by huge fear. Handled incorrectly, more harm than good could be done to her. I suggested I give her a Reiki treatment, which I assured her was soothing and relaxing and would reveal nothing to me.

I knew there was something significant going on with her, so, under guidance of Spirit and with full protection in place, I scanned her energy field as I worked. I could clearly see where her problems originated. She had been sexually abused as a child. There were enough bruises in various stages of healing to suggest that her husband had started physically abusing her. So often the original wounding replays itself in our lives giving us an opportunity to make different choices. I understood that forcing her to admit to what she was hiding could cause more harm than good. Her only aim at this stage was to test the waters.

I worked with her for many months before she decided she felt worthy of being saved and became brave enough to see a therapist. Giving her Reiki treatments soothed her and while she was relaxing, I worked with her blocked chakras to get some energy flowing through her shut down system. I connected her to her Upstairs team to allow them to begin working with her.

She was aware of none of this. She simply thought she was having a Reiki treatment which she found unthreatening. Slowly she began to feel stronger and she began to open up and talk to me about her desire to make changes in her life. She never told me what was going on at home. I focussed on her sense of well-being, not her problems. To throw her in the deep end would have sent her scuttling back into hiding and I needed to work gently with her. We worked on simple things like introducing a short daily walk (physical body). Singing in the shower (emotional body) although the best she could do was to hum.

I lent her a copy of the *Tao of Pooh* (mental body) as there really is the most beautiful wisdom in the world of Winnie the Pooh. What she perceived as childish philosophy didn't threaten her. Finally, for her spiritual body I had her spend a few minutes twice a day sitting quietly in the bathroom, where she felt safe, saying an affirmation quietly to herself. She didn't manage to look herself in the eye in the mirror while she practiced her affirmations, but she did them resolutely as suggested.

With her focus being gently redirected towards self-care, she began to find a sense of herself again. One day she very bravely said to me, "I have something really dreadful to tell you." I didn't allow her to tell me her story. I was not qualified to deal with her violent domestic situation and she needed specialist help. I reassured her that I knew she was going through something significant and I gave her the name of three different professionals that I knew could work with her.

She seemed relieved and I suggested that I remain a safe space where she could come outside of her situation, just to have her tanks refilled as it were, a space to be gentled. Therapy can rock your world especially when dealing with such significant issues. I believe that supportive treatments, therapies and measures are an important part of achieving success in the long term. It was a long road, but she succeeded in leaving her abusive husband and she moved overseas. Whether she ever addressed her childhood abuse I do not know. Upstairs clearly showed me that it was not part of my mandate to work with. I have to honour that.

I appear to have digressed again. Back to our bathtub reflection. Next on the agenda is your mental self. Have you learned anything new recently? Have you applied your knowledge in a useful way? Have you allowed your intuition a voice, and more importantly, have you applied what it might be telling you? Your physical self can literally remove you from an unbalanced situation, your emotional self might react to it, but your mental body is how you can think yourself into or out of it, using knowledge or instinct. Here's the place where, on reflection, you might decide to study something, read a book, learn a new language, or just spend time in solitude thinking something through. There is always some small incremental change one can make mentally that could end up having a profound effect on your life.

Finally, have a look at your spiritual self. That doesn't necessarily interpret as did you go to church or temple, meditate or do yoga, although these are all good practices. It means how have you honoured yourself. Have you acknowledged all that you are and offered gratitude to yourself for all that you have achieved in life, or conversely how you have survived thus far in life? Making changes to your spiritual well-being can be as simple as taking a nap or sitting quietly just being with yourself with no demands and no expectations. It might be a walk on the beach or listening to an inspirational podcast or it might be a thirty second happy dance. It is about finding your joy, your bliss, and celebrating it.

The last step in your bathtub reflection is to step out of the water all shiny new and clean. You have a solid plan with easily achievable goals and you are set for success. You pull the plug and any negativity you may have acknowledged, is whooshed away down the plug hole. You get to start again with a clean slate for tomorrow unencumbered and unburdened. Until your next reflection. Always commit to being honest with yourself. Honesty over judgement.

The beauty about all of these practices is that it is your own reflection of your own journey. It is not open to the distorted interpretations of anyone else. No one's opinion truly matters other than your own. If you are happy and fulfilled in your life, content and at peace, then it is nobody's business to try and change you or move you out of your comfort zone.

However, once you do register a genuine desire for change, there is so much that you can do for yourself. If you get stuck, or you cannot motivate yourself to carry out the changes you've identified, remember that you can always harness the services of professionals. There are many disciplines available to choose from. Personally, I have found coaching to be extremely useful when making changes in life. The professional body has much learning and often great wisdom to offer you that you may not be privy to.

Be wary however, of those who seek to tell you what you should do. You are then being subjected to their interpretation of your stories as seen through their filters. Even then, they can still be very useful for gaining new perspectives, but it remains wholly and completely your choice to embrace, respond to, react to, or reject their counsel. Only you can make a lasting change to your life. At any stage you retain the right to change again and again and again, until you come to a place of understanding and peace and you are living a life focussed on joy.

Chapter 45

Setting boundaries

By this stage I had admitted to myself that my way of life was a problem for me. I had finally decided to do something about it. I had sought council from all and sundry and I had decided to make some pretty big changes in my life. I had deep dived into the scary dark places in my mind and had overturned enough rocks to let the light in. I was seeing life more clearly at this point than ever before. The changes in me were really significant and I was desperate to cling to those changes and not revert back to my usual fear and unworthiness... and yes I do know that the desperation I just referred to is a fear based term!

One of the most important things we can learn to do when making changes in our lives is to set boundaries. Naturally I completely misunderstood the concept of boundaries. I experienced every boundary through the filters of my own unworthiness. My whole life I had accepted every boundary and limit from every source, as I had been taught to do just to survive my own upbringing. It was never a problem for me... until it became a problem.

With every layer of my life that I peeled back, wrestled with and healed; and with every part of me I recovered as I did my journey work, I began to perceive the world in a different way. Change always comes with consequences. For the most part the consequences are a better, more comfortable relationship with yourself, a lighter, happier way of living your life. Through the years of living inauthentically, I had collected and gathered around me a cast of characters who were engaged to either teach me what I needed to learn, or who would trigger me again and again until I finally found my way back to my true sense of self.

I was quite appalled at how easy it seemed to be for so many people in my life to treat me really disrespectfully. Clearly, I had set a very bad example of my worth. Setting boundaries is a powerful way to protect your new way of being until such time as it becomes a new natural instinct. Boundaries show the world where your tolerance levels end and they send out a clear message as to how you expect to be treated.

Since I was the one who had changed, it seemed only fair that I should be the one to set some boundaries. Having never had any boundaries before, this proved to be challenging. However, when we change our life strategies, we need to change our behaviour to support our new way of being and one of those behaviours is boundary setting. It was no coincidence that at this stage in my life the boundary setters showed up in their droves to teach me what I needed to learn. I did a great casting job when I built this life plan.

If you think about it, behind every behaviour, there is a feeling or an emotion acting as a driving force. What I have come to understand is that underneath every feeling or emotion, is a need for love in one or all of its glorious distortions. Perhaps we did not feel loved during our formative years and we learned to act out in order to be seen, to attract attention. Maybe we have been loved to the point of entitlement and we keep demanding more and more love to validate our state of being.

So often we lash out in anger because although we inherently understand that we have the right to be loved, our life experiences have deprived us of love, leaving us feeling unworthy and hard done by; and so we act out our frustration and our pain. Often, we are so filled with self-loathing through the distortions of love we have experienced, we act in and we hurt ourselves either by substance abuse, cutting, sexual deviance or by aligning ourselves with groups who are only too happy to give us negative attention. Or perhaps we act out by becoming people pleasing doormats and allowing the world to use us at will regardless of how we feel about it. There are as many permutations of this state as there are distortions of love.

I first experienced boundaries in a very negative way. As a newcomer to living an authentic life, I found boundaries terribly limiting and frustrating. As with all new ways of being I had hopelessly overcorrected and become a one-woman vigilante on my own behalf. I quickly found myself knocking up against other people's boundaries and I felt edited, disempowered and disallowed. Dismantling an emotional trigger can sometimes be a complex multi-layered business. At times the simple act of acknowledging a trigger and shining some light on it, can be sufficient to disconnect it, especially when coupled with a strong desire for change. Other more complex triggers, may need to be dismantled and broken down into a range of smaller less powerful triggers to be dealt with separately, before you can release yourself from their control. The truly tough ones might need the energetic equivalent of a bomb disposal unit to break them down, and until you finally make your peace with yourself they cling like limpet mines. Boundaries and mindfulness are your greatest allies when dealing with this last category.

This is why all my old learnings and pain leapt to the forefront again and I spiralled back into confusion and self-doubt. I stumbled into a boundary, felt triggered and I became frozen by indecision. Did I have the right to challenge someone else's boundary, especially if it was hurting me? Why were my old patterns of thinking looming so large again? Hadn't I dealt with that? I felt like the living embodiment of the expression damned if I do, and damned if I don't. Having freed myself from the dictates of the inner voices of other people, and having found my own inner voice, I seemed to be falling at the first hurdle… the boundaries. I had no idea how to respect a boundary or how to create one. I found them paralysing.

There is a simple explanation for why it is so difficult to escape the old trauma patterns in your life. Living a trauma-based life requires high levels of chaos to sustain it. Without chaos, trauma cannot express itself. When we are in the throes of our dysfunctional, unbalanced, or non-authentic existence, we are living in a trauma vortex. If you can picture a funnel then you will understand what I mean. You are at the bottom of the funnel in the narrowest part and the trauma and chaos is almost constant as it swirls around in your energy field. As you begin to heal, your vibration raises and you lift higher up the funnel. Here's where I need to challenge a paradigm. We think time is a linear construct when in actual fact it is cyclical in nature, which is why as you raise yourself out of the chaos of your trauma-based life, the same old problems and triggers keep coming around albeit with less frequency. The higher you raise your vibration the wider the mouth of the funnel, and the longer intervals between each occurrence becomes. Why is this so? Well, since energy cannot be destroyed and since those significant events that imprinted themselves with such force that they essentially changed who you were, cannot be made to vanish, they will always be a part of your story. However, with every healing pass you make, you transmute the pain associated with those circumstances out of shadow and into the light and you relieve the pressure of the connection. Much like when you press the little weights on a pressure cooker to relieve the pressure and prevent it from exploding; so too you transmute the pressure build-up from your personal triggers and release the accompanying charge. With enough conscious effort you will get to the point where you will recognise your old triggers as they come around, yet again, but you will be able to stand still and breathe as they pass you by without any charge at all. That is what it means to be healed.

Harnessing my old fail-safe method of read, research, explore and question, I came to realise that any change to lifelong learning, requires a lot of patience and repetitive, continual practice to develop into a new natural instinct. As with anything you learn, repetition is the only path to expertise. My new way of thinking and my new beliefs in my innate right to be fully me were fledgling feelings. I had not yet learned to be instinctively me, so when I ran across a boundary and it triggered me, my old default setting kicked in, the old ingrained worthless me. I learned that only through mindful attention to my responses could I change how I behaved. I needed conscious practice.

I may well continue to be triggered by people and commentary that I perceive to be limiting or threatening to me. But, with mindful attention to my responses and, more critically, by practising a momentary pause between trigger and response, I can learn to choose my reaction and thus manage my behaviour. The fact that I still feel triggered, simply indicates that there is unresolved latent pain that hasn't been fully healed. By managing my emotional responses and redirecting my actions in a manner that is congruent with my new way of being, I can begin to lay down new pathways in my brain and I can build new instincts. At some point, through conscious effort and compassionate awareness, I will no longer take the old dusty off-road tracks that I learned to travel as a small child, and continued on for most of my life, I can take the on ramp to the super-highway of consciousness.

Having finally understood boundaries, I set some of my own. It is important to note that a boundary isn't about demanding or expecting others to change their behaviours. Boundaries should also never be punitive in nature, that might be construed as bullying. They are about you deciding to limit your exposure to harmful influences or situations incongruent with your way of being, or your comfort.

This is the reason that newly clean and sober addicts are cautioned not to hang out with their former drinking or drugging buddies. Until their sobriety becomes ingrained, after lots and lots of practice, they are too vulnerable to fend off the intoxicatingly inviting world of their previous soothing and calming methods. Having exposed their wounds and made new choices, they are very vulnerable to relapse. It becomes a moral imperative to limit triggering situations and people, until they are more soundly entrenched and grounded in their new way of being. Insert your wounding in the place of addiction and the requirements are the same.

This doesn't mean you have to remove yourself from society or lock yourself away in a safe space just to cope; it means you need to treat yourself with the utmost respect and give yourself the best possible chance at succeeding in your new way of being. Remember energy flows where thought goes and as you begin to heal, a healthy response when you feel triggered is to pause. Consider what it was that triggered you. Acknowledge the emotion and the need behind the feelings.

Breathe until you are clear of your old story and autopilot response. Then decide how you want to proceed. Be mindful of not putting your energy into anything that doesn't expressly add value to your life. The more you surround yourself with situations, people and influences that support your way of being, the easier it will be for you to entrench your new behaviours; the quicker you can build those new natural instincts.

I love the analogy of teaching a child to swim when I think about living in a new way. Children learn how to walk and run and jump and climb, but suddenly you require them to learn to swim. They have no instinctive responses to draw from in the water and they need to learn how to manage in this new environment.

You wouldn't throw a small child into the deep end of the pool and tell them to sink or swim. You would go into the water with them. You would give them flotation aids. You would support their little bodies until they became comfortable in the water. Then you would teach them the skills needed to stay afloat and most critically... how to get themselves out of the water. Then, and only then, when their safety is assured, do you teach them how to swim the various strokes and styles. Small incremental steps with loads of safety measures in place... that is the role of a boundary, they are safety measures to protect your way of being.

Boundaries can also be used inappropriately. My friend was angry with me when she thought I had been lying to her about my health for over thirty years, and she put down a boundary to punish me for what she perceived was a transgression of the highest order on my part. I understand why she did this, but because her boundary was hurting me, I believe I had the right to challenge it. I came to this realisation too late to save the friendship, but then aren't so many of our greatest insights found by looking backwards.

I have another acquaintance who has some very serious issues in her life that threaten her well-being and safety. She is fully conscious of this and is in no way, shape or form prepared to make any changes to support a new way of being. She starves herself and refuses to eat properly. She thinks it makes her beautiful, youthful and attractive which is what her wounding tells her she needs to be in order to be acceptable and lovable. In reality she is gaunt, unhealthy and haggard, she is the picture of self-neglect. However, it simply hasn't become a big enough problem yet for her to want to change. Any attempts to help or guide her are met with ghosting behaviour. She simply removes herself from anyone who questions her choices – she puts a boundary between herself and anyone wishing to help her. Her boundary protects her way of being and is a very effective way of making sure nothing gets through.

I worked with another client who was being verbally abused by her husband. She needed help so desperately, but it had to be on her terms, All I could do was to provide her with a safe space to be and we spent many months just sitting quietly together not discussing her problems until she finally decided she wanted to change.

No one has the right to try to change you, or to save you, or to make you different in any way, unless, and until, you ask for help. This is why people who are forced to go into rehab have a greater chance of failure and relapse than those who are ready and wanting to make a change to a new way of being. Change cannot be forced on someone who is not willing to make the necessary changes to their actions and behaviours to support a different existence.

Having lived on the edge of fear and in a constant state of disempowerment, being battered by situations I had no ability to affect, I found I was very susceptible to fear energy. I decided to no longer allow myself to be inundated with the brutality and disaster stories on social media. I do not read newspapers, nor will I watch the news on television. When people tell me, breathless with fear, about the latest mass casualty tragedy or destruction taking place, or the latest social campaign against terror and abuse, I do not become involved.

I am not unsympathetic to the causes and I will happily sit in meditation and pour calming, healing energy out to the victims of an earthquake or a mass shooting. I will not, however, sit and build on the fear that goes with the social discourse on such matters. The last thing the victims of these events need is a mass outpouring of fear and negative energy. They have generated more than their fair share of such emotions already and to have them amplified across the globe extends and exacerbates their feelings of shock and trauma.

If one cannot be a first responder, or part of a team to physically assist, or to help in any meaningful way, then it is better to send focussed healing and calming energies in their direction. Hold the space of the base, heart, crown so that they can still their fear and panic and can begin to make sense of their new reality. Let them feel your outpouring of love and support, not your fear and your anger.

If you look on a global scale, economic sanctions are a wonderful example of boundary setting. Countries who perpetrated behaviours unacceptable to their trade partners were slapped with economic sanctions. This was a message that said very clearly, we do not support your way of being and to protect our way of being we will remove ourselves from any contact with you, and we will no longer reward you with our favour and business.

All change comes with consequences and it is up to each party to decide for themselves whether the consequences of that boundary is something they can live with or not. If it made their way of being uncomfortable enough that it became a problem for them, then perhaps they might have been stirred to find another way of being. An economic sanction does not insist that the other party change, but it certainly has the effect of giving them a new consequence to consider. It is up to the sanctioned country to decide if it wants to change or not.

With the new rise of feminine energy, women's empowerment issues are a hot topic across the globe. I remember with distinct discomfort the #MeToo campaign that raised the lid on the Pandora's box of sexual harassment and misconduct across the world. Many shocking revelations were made and some horrendous stories were shared. Sadly, some heinous lies were also told by women with anger issues and hidden agendas unrelated to the subject (unhealed wounds).

In this instance it was quite overwhelming to hear previously silenced women roar publicly and unapologetically, finding their voices after years of suppression and silence. I do not know one single woman in my orbit who either didn't have her own #Story or who didn't know someone else who did. This was a magnificent example of boundary setting. Women across the globe banded together in solidarity and set a collective boundary letting all men know in no uncertain terms where their tolerance levels ended, and precisely how they expected to be treated going forward.

Has it solved the problem? Probably not, but what it has done is made women less afraid to speak up. That in turn has a restraining effect on perpetrators because there is now a very real possibility that they will be outed and publicly named and shamed… they will experience a new consequence. It is a small, yet significant step in healing the sexual inequalities inherent in our society.

All change comes with consequence and another offshoot of the #MeToo campaign is that men are feeling victimised. The good guys who do not sexually harass their colleagues, students, partners or subordinates are crying out that they have been tarnished with the same brush and they are hurting. They are being told that their identity is no longer acceptable in the eyes of the feminine. Given that we are moving into a new feminine energy era, I can understand how this would create fear and instability for the good guys.

The pendulum has swung in the opposite direction and we have transferred the disempowerment to the other side. Two wrongs have never, in the history of the world, made a right and I'm certain there will be a knock-on effect from this in the future. I absolutely respect your right to disagree with me on this and any other opinion I have, and I will recognise your point of view and reserve the right to disagree with you in turn. Time will tell all.

This, for me, highlights the problem with mass generalisations. Generalisations can lead to huge misunderstanding and that in turn has the effect of raising fear and anger and can even lead to the inciting of violence. I am guilty of generalisation. I do it to highlight a point or to make something complex more easily understandable. I do not do it to foster separateness. I believe that if we focus on separateness then we create that very condition. That is extremely undesirable and is counter-productive to the improving and uplifting of humanity.

I also recognise that the recipients of my generalisations may not perceive what I am saying in the manner I intended, because their filters are different to mine. They will hear my generalisations through the filters created by their life experiences and there is great risk of distortion. It is no wonder then that we see twitchy, over-sensitive powder keg ready to explode type responses on social media posts. The reactions are based on each individual's history with trauma and it stands to reason that miscommunication and misunderstandings are rife.

It is incumbent upon each of us to articulate a better argument to support our message. We need to find a way to make ourselves stronger/heard/respected/great, without standing on someone else's head to make our point. The clinging together in fear, I find most disempowering. Mass campaigns focussed on love, togetherness and positivity are needed to build and foster the energy of change and respect.

South Africa is a country with a turbulent social situation. We exist in a post-apartheid era where atrocities of the past have yet to be fully healed. There is so much imbalance in the way South Africans experience life. We have so much separateness still as we struggle to find a way to fully mesh our society into one collective. We still do not speak as one voice and fear abounds. A social media campaign has been launched called #I'mStaying. This group is open to all layers of South African society and its members share stories of hope and togetherness. They share their positive experiences as South Africans and I find it heart-warming. People from diverse backgrounds, cultures and communities share their stories and their commitment to a better future for our rainbow nation. Since energy flows where thought goes, I am personally very excited to see this initiative gain momentum as we begin to focus our energy on the kind of future that we want to live in.

I am personally very clear on one point and I will repeat it over and over again in spite of the negative reception I so often get when I say it. There is only one thing that you have any jurisdiction over in this lifetime, only one thing you have any control over, or any right to change… and that is your own actions and responses. I believe with every fibre of my being that if we each took care of our own well-being, worked on healing our own wounds, we would be able to engage with our fellow man in a more authentic, balanced manner and there would be such an intense rise in the collective consciousness that our planet would begin to heal. It can be done.

Chapter 46

Belonging

I was sitting in an Inner Tuition class one day and I was feeling particularly at sea. My health was shocking. I could no longer work, my days of identifying as a mother were over, my daughters had flown the nest and were responsible for their own lives. I didn't have a personal relationship. I had lost my home, my dog, my independence. I was back living with my ex and I wasn't in a great space emotionally. I was struggling with the realisation that my mother had wished I had never been born and I hadn't yet made my peace with that revelation. My world had been rocked off its axis, I had lost one of my oldest and dearest friends and I was hopelessly lost.

I was co-facilitating a new course at the request of the facilitator and I was listening to her introduce the new batch of students. This is so and so, she's an accountant, this one is a lawyer, this one is a nurse, a psychologist, a florist... and that's Janice. Just that. Nothing else. Nothing to recommend me or to show the students I had any standing in the eyes of the facilitator, or indeed the world. Nothing to contribute, nothing to add. I felt so undermined and worthless I wondered why I was even there.

I have been a bank clerk; a medical technologist; a real estate agent, I've run a home industry; been a personal assistant; I've done print and production; been a contact centre agent; a catalogue manager; a copywriter; I've been a facilities manager; I've managed an online shopping mall; I've been a toastmaster; an ISO auditor; a business analyst; a tarot reader; a psychic; an energetic intuitive; an Inner Tuition facilitator; a Reiki practitioner; a Quantum Genius operator, I've worked in a rehabilitation centre; I'm an author; a designer, and so much more besides. But none of that seemed worthy of being mentioned.

I'm surprised I didn't scare the students away, because I cried almost all the way through the sixteen-week course. I was strong when it came to disseminating information and explaining the often brand-new concepts to the students. I had a knack for being able to distil pages of information down into bite size nuggets that could be easily digested. I could hold the energy in the room and I knew how to support a student who might be struggling. I worked with great empathy for their journeys, for I knew first-hand just how difficult it could be to deal with some of the things that came into consciousness on these journeys of discovery. However, when it came time for the practical exercises and I tapped into my own inner journey, the world dissolved around me as I struggled with my demons.

My pain, when viewed from outside may not have seemed significant to others, but in my heart and soul it was paralysing. I was told over and over again throughout the course what I *just needed to do*, but I couldn't hear it. My pain and despair had made me unreceptive, and all I heard was condescension. I knew that my journey had been hard, very hard indeed. I had been beaten down to within an inch of my life on so many occasions and to be told in a tone, that to my ears inferred I was stupid, that I *just needed to...*

Now I am not an unintelligent woman, nor am I unaware. I had spent decades struggling to find answers. I know for a fact that if the solutions were that simple, I would have *just found* them years ago. I felt dismissed, marginalised, unvalidated when I longed for empathy, understanding and comfort. I longed for a community and a place where I felt accepted and supported and valued. I had lost my work community. I was still in touch with only three or four of my colleagues. Over twenty years of relationships vaporised as though they had never existed. I simply no longer appeared to have any value given that I didn't work somewhere or do something impressive. I had no degree or qualification to hide behind. I voiced over and over my need for a sense of belonging and acceptance, a place to hang my hat. I bared my tortured soul and always the answer was the same, *you just need to…*

I still felt like that tiny baby desperate to be held. I closed myself off in a prison of my own making and the filters of my past distorted all sounds. I heard dismissive, patronising condescension, where in reality I was being given support and encouragement. I really wanted to run away, to leave the course, but I stayed because I had made a commitment to the students. You can see how deep in despair I was. Nothing made any sense to me as I swirled around in a miasma of pain and misery.

Then one day the facilitator brought out a document and began to read. She said, "Greetings from Home dear ones." It was a transcript of a channelled message and as she read it, every word spoke directly to my heart. It was as if the letter had been written to me personally. It spoke of how we belong to a vast spiritual family and we are here on Earth playing the game of humanity. We wrote the rules for the game and the way our game here on Earth differs from all other games, is that we are the only planet where people have free will. It has been a source of great interest to all the others in the celestial realm, to see how we play our game here on Earth. The channel spoke of how amazed they were at our capacity for suffering.

As humans, if we found ourselves in a difficult or uncomfortable situation, we didn't automatically make a different decision and find a more comfortable way of living, no, we adapted and we found a way to live with the discomfort. This is something Upstairs are quite astounded by. It is not congruent with a joyful existence and it puzzles them greatly. They are however, so proud of the job we are doing and they reminded us that each of us has a specific role to play and that none of us are here at this time by mistake. Apparently, what is happening on Earth right now is the equivalent of a celestial Super Bowl final and we are being cheered along with great alacrity. Suddenly everything became clear and I remembered who I was and why I was here.

If you do as I did and you research channelled messages, you will find a wealth of information on the subject from many different sources. I read as much of that particular channel as I could find and many others besides. Once again, when I scrubbed the messages down to the bare bones and identified the similarities, here is what I discovered. I finally understood that what happens here on Earth is not the end game, it is a small part of a much bigger game we are playing. I belong to a Celestial family, I am a Spiritual being, and I am a part of this multi-facetted game called Humanity whereby the great Creator, the All that is, is experiencing every facet of itself. As all the players in the game achieve enlightenment, along the many levels of the game, humanity will reach its full potential and all of life will finally be... as it is in Heaven.

The channels speak of changes being made to the game, of a need to escalate the learning. Earth's resources have been stretched and mismanaged and some changes need to be affected if we are to survive. To that end there has been a thinning of the veil between our world and beyond making it easier for human beings to access their memories, their original plans, their project teams. Humanity can now access, with greater ease, the knowledge required to play out our allotted roles. Everyone has a specific piece of the puzzle and only by attaining our own enlightenment, can we place our specific puzzle piece in the game. With each piece placed, it becomes easier and easier for the souls following us to find their way too. We are charged with laying bread crumb trails for others to help them stay on course.

The chaos in our social structure today is simply as a result of the changes taking place on our planet. We are moving away from a controlling, dominant, masculine energy into a feminine energy phase or cycle, as it were. The feminine energy is more supporting and nurturing and this is a time where humanity needs to open their collective hearts. The increase in the gender neutrality issues, the differently abled children, syndrome illnesses, all aspects of humanity that challenge the social status quo, are all opportunities for humanity to learn to love itself in all of its many guises.

Tolerance is no longer an acceptable goal. Our challenge is to fully and completely accept all aspects of ourselves as a shared humanity. We are *Spiritual* beings having a *Human* experience through the medium of *Love.* Everything in between that framework is dependent on the choices we make along the way. I believe it is critical to this mission that we understand the following: we do not have to agree on a single thing to treat one another with kindness.

Chapter 47

So what now?

Life can be so ironic. I finally made my peace with my childhood. I finally removed all of my masks. I no longer need to hide who I am, because I fully understand that other people's opinions of me are truly none of my business. I am, at last, at peace with the fact that my happiness is a choice I get to make on a daily basis. I no longer wake up and test my body to see what kind of a day I'm going to be allowed to have. I wake up and yes, I still register pain on most days, but I then *decide* what kind of a day I want to have.

If I need a rest day, I take one and I focus on being grateful for being able to rest when I need to. I use that down time to expand my learning. I read, I listen to podcasts and if necessary, I allow myself to sleep. I no longer yearn for things I have lost, but rather I celebrate the memories I have of the joy I felt at those times when I had so much available to me. I have fewer friends and I only expend energy on those with whom I resonate. Judgemental, self-involved, draining people are no longer a match for my energy and I am careful about where I spend my time and who I spend it with.

I have also discovered that self-care is an absolutely prerequisite to my being able to live this way. Overextend myself physically or energetically, spend time around people not in synch with my energy and I pay the price. I go right back into a state of exhaustion and chaos and all my old demons pop in for a visit. Each time it is easier for me to regain resonance and clarity and I draw my boundaries tighter and learn how to support myself properly by engaging in activities that foster joy and well-being.

I decided I would completely give up on searching for a diagnosis and I would simply focus my energy on maximising my joy within each day that I have, with whatever means I have at my disposal. And here's where the irony comes in. I went to see a kinesiologist I had consulted maybe ten or twelve years ago. I went to him to see if I still held any limiting beliefs in my energy field. He's fully into the weird shit that I love so much and I was confident he would unearth anything still hiding, that needed some light shone on it. He was terribly surprised to say that he could find nothing that I needed to work on. It was extremely rare to come across someone who has done all of their work. I felt quite proud of myself. I had worked really hard on my recovery and having achieved what I considered an emotional sobriety, I was thrilled to have it acknowledged. He did, however, say that on a physical level I had a number of health syndromes that needed to be dealt with. The two main ones would be tackled first.

One was SIBO, a small intestinal bacterial overgrowth. The small intestines become flooded with bacteria that should only ever be located in the large intestine. If you research this condition you will find that it ticks the boxes of almost eighty percent of my symptoms, including Vitamin B12 and iron deficiencies (low ferritin), inability to absorb food due to damage caused to the intestinal lining, abdominal bloating and pain, decreased fat absorption leading to Vitamin A and D deficiencies, food allergies and sensitivities, chronic fatigue, body pain, burdened liver, fatigue after exertion, hypothyroid, and excretion by bacteria of high amounts of acids leading to neurological and cognitive symptoms. He felt that two to three months of treatment should be sufficient to bring this under control.

The second syndrome I needed to tackle was Lyme disease! I told him I had tested negative for Rickettsia although positive for past exposure to many of the co-infections. He confirmed that only three percent of Lyme Disease is actually picked up by laboratory tests. He had no doubt at all that this was what was wrong with me and what had plagued me for most of my adult life. He recommended treatment for eight to twelve months including daily use of the Rife machine. He is confident that after a year, nearly all of my symptoms would have gone.

I sat with this information for a few days and tried to decide how I felt about it. Whichever way I looked at it, I couldn't seem to get too worked up about it. I realised I no longer needed to identify with a diagnosis. I didn't need to validate my suffering for anyone else. I was living a life focussed on my own joy and happiness and my goal was to live with an open heart. I decided I would take the treatment, experience the side effects, and work my way around to jolly good health, or not, however it turns out. I have paddled around in the murky depths of the medical fountain for years with absolutely no results. Now I am going to embrace the alternative and the weird shit and give it a go. If it works, fabulous. If it doesn't then I haven't lost anything by trying and I shall be no worse off for the effort.

I have started a small design business called Sticky Corners. I design photobooks for people and I have found the projects to have such spirit and to be so evocative. I have done celebrations of ninety-year olds, granny brag books, travel memories, family trees, wedding celebrations, birthdays and so many other special occasions, fur babies and pet's albums, and I have even done the occasional thesis presentation in a creative manner. I took my sister's photographs of her years sailing round the world with her late partner and I made her a beautiful coffee table book with those precious memories. That chapter in her life was closed symbolically with the closing of the book. The next chapter is up to her to write, whenever she feels ready.

I've written my children's book, Warthog Tales, and I have shared that joyous experience with the world. I thought about getting a new dog and I had almost convinced myself that a new dog would motivate me to get out and exercise. In reality motivation has never really been my problem since I love to exercise. Pain and weakness are my problems. I made an unplanned stop at the same spiritual fair where I had received word from my sister's late partner. I queued up to see the same psychic and this time he told me that a large black dog had stepped forward. He described him as a pitch-black Scooby Doo dog. Scooby Doo is a Great Dane. I was stunned. Was this my beautiful boy?

The psychic then made a reference to the dog leaning up against a fridge with his head on one side as if to indicate a strange noise. I had said to ex-Husband the previous evening that the fridge was making an odd noise and I thought we should get it checked out. He then said to me that he knew I was thinking of getting a new dog and he urged me not to do it. He said I wasn't strong enough and the time was not right. When the time was right, my precious boy would ensure that the right companion would come to me.

I had a rough winter. I had three bouts of flu back to back, each one tougher to bear than the last. I was in a bad way. My eardrums were bulging, my sinuses were clogged and swollen, my throat was on fire, my chest was as tight as a drum, I ran a high fever, I had vertigo, I was nauseous and vomiting and I felt as through my brain was on fire. It was impossible to keep my eyes open or to sit up. I lurched from one pain injection to the next and in desperation, I contacted my friend at Inner Tuition and begged her to intercede with upstairs on my behalf.

She duly did and the message came back loud and clear. We have been downloading information into your brain and you have done nothing with it. It is causing your ears to bulge and is putting pressure on your brain. If you want to feel better, you need to start writing. It's time for you to do what you are here to do and to prepare your piece of the puzzle. Who am I to argue with a celestial instruction from Home?

Epilogue

I really hope I haven't come across as a whiny, self-indulgent victim. I am nothing of the sort. I hid an extraordinary life from everyone I knew, for reasons I didn't fully understand and I lost myself in the process. The harder I yearned to be ordinary, the more I seemed to drive it away from me. I have subsequently learned through reading about the Law of Attraction from many sources, that if you spend your energy wanting to attract something into your life, then that is exactly what you attract… the wanting. The way to be ordinary is to celebrate your ordinariness in much the same way as I celebrated my trip to Mauritius. I didn't focus on wanting to win, I told everyone how amazing it was going to be when I got there and I focussed on the joy.

I no longer desire to be ordinary. I am quite content being the unique soul that I am. My true home is on the other side of that ever-thinning veil, and there I am celebrated indeed. Celebrated here on Earth? Perhaps not, but that isn't what's important. This is only the game that I am playing. The cast of characters who have littered my journey thus far, have done their jobs well. I have learned so much from all of them, even if some of the lessons were very painful. I am delighted to continue sharing my experience with so many of you and I eagerly anticipate our adventures together.

Having now exposed myself and my weird-shit philosophies and thinking, I am fully aware that I may lose more people from my life as I evolve and become incongruent with their way of being. For those souls, our time together may be done here on Earth, but I look forward to meeting up with you on the other side where there is no judgement and there is only love. I can no longer pretend to be invisible and mould myself to the expectations and needs of others to gain acceptance. All change comes with consequences and I needed to change to survive. I also look forward to meeting any new characters I have written into my life plan for the future and I wonder what we shall get up to together.

I was gifted a reading with a medium I had not met before and it was incredible that so many of the characters who had been in my life raced in to greet me. My in-laws came to say how sorry they were that they had been so hard on me. My Dad came through, again telling me how beautiful the gardens are on the other side. He is with Mother and they are so happy. My beautiful Great Dane is with them and they adore him. My darling dog thanked me for that last outing to the beach and for the photographs I have of him in my home and he said how much he loved me.

I met my maternal grandmother. Mother was adopted and I knew nothing about her family. She identified herself as Lily and she said she works with me when I am doing healing work. She spoke about being with me at the time when my car was stolen and she mentioned a number of other very private details that as far as I know, no one is privy to. And finally, Mother came to me. Her name was Daisy Jane Beatrice, but we knew her as Betty. She came through with the name Daisy. Her energy was warm and comfortable and somehow familiar although, not at all what I knew from her time here on Earth.

She said that she is now well and whole and happy. She said that her mental illness had made me become very hard on myself and that had had a knock-on effect my whole life through. She said she was so sorry for how she had treated me. She also said that on the other side there is no pain or judgement and one sees things with so much more clarity. She referenced a ring she had given me. It was the one act of Mother's that made me feel connected to her in any meaningful way.

When she had worn it, the ring was set with a ruby and as a little girl I loved to try it on and pretend I was a grown up. She had reset it with an amethyst, my birth stone, and had given it to me for a birthday. It was stolen one day when my house was burgled and she acknowledged how sad that had made me. Then for the first time she said the following words, "I really do love you." I had waited my whole life to hear those words. I asked her how she felt about me writing this story and she said it was necessary and she fully supported it.

If I have written anything in this book that resonates with even one person; and helps them to find their way back to their true self, then my work here is done and I am happy to have been of service. Remember it doesn't matter how far off track you get in life, there is always time to redirect yourself. Nothing changes until you change it and that starts with a desire to have a different experience. Good luck finding whatever it is that lights you up in this crazy life and then share that light with everyone you meet.

Be the light in your own life first and foremost. Remember too, that it truly isn't what has happened to you, or even what might still be happening beyond your control, that is of importance, what is important is what you do with it, what you learn from it and how you respond to it. The critical element to bringing change to your life is to manage the way you respond to your emotional triggers. If you can figure that out, you will have found your power. If you are toting around unhealed wounds you will continue to be triggered, take offense and feel afraid. Not one single person has the right to treat you badly and I urge you to be your own greatest advocate.

Whilst nothing is really a problem, until it becomes a real problem for you, do remember that your body and your soul are desperately seeking resonance in all things. If your body is showing you something, please listen. If you are unhappy and frustrated in life, go within. If you can, still your mind and quieten your inner critic long enough to identify and commune with your authentic self; find out if that inner voice that is directing your life is the voice of your own true self, or of someone else you unknowingly gave your power over to; you will find the answers you seek. With every part of yourself that you can reclaim, you will lessen the emotional charge, disconnect the triggers and you'll find you are no longer controlled by your out-of-control responses. You will be able to move through your pain, break unhealthy patterns, and you can begin to write the next chapter of your story in line with your heart's desire.

Above all don't be afraid of the weird shit. Different doesn't always translate as dangerous. Some of the most incredible gifts I ever received in life came wrapped in the weirdest of guises. There comes a point in life where you are compelled through the onboarding of new knowledge to be a different version of yourself. Once I became curious enough to be bold enough to take a closer look, my journey took on an extraordinary slant. My mind and thinking were blown wide open and the kernels of wisdom and insights I gained have set me on a whole new path in life.

I finally found my light and the courage to let it shine.

Made in the USA
Monee, IL
13 September 2026

62976613R00148